THE
FITNESS CURRENCY

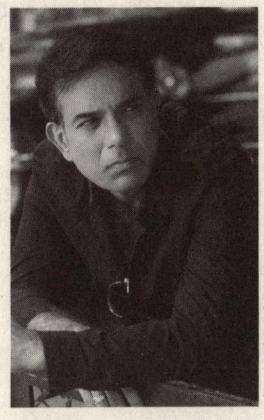

Utkarsh Rai is a management consultant and coach. He is a former Managing Director of Infinera India. A recipient of Udyog Rattan Award, he is the author of two popular books: *Faster Smarter Higher: Managing Your Career* and *101 Myths and Realities @ the Office*.

From being massively overweight to regaining fitness, Utkarsh is an inspiration for many. He is also an angel investor in start-ups. His hobbies include acting and travelling to offbeat destinations.

Praise for the book

The Prime Minister always says that our professional workforce is the engine that drives the economy and their fitness is critical to enable them to give their best. Weaving fitness into their busy lifestyle is the key to growth. #HumFitTohIndiaFit

—Col Rajyavardhan Rathore, AVSM (Retd),
Minister of Youth Affairs &
Sports and Information & Broadcasting

THE
FITNESS CURRENCY

AT ANY STAGE
AT ANY AGE

UTKARSH RAI

Published by
Rupa Publications India Pvt. Ltd 2018
7/16, Ansari Road, Daryaganj
New Delhi 110002

Sales centres:

Allahabad Bengaluru Chennai
Hyderabad Jaipur Kathmandu
Kolkata Mumbai

Copyright © Utkarsh Rai 2018

While every effort has been made to verify the authenticity of the information contained in this book, the publisher and the author are in no way liable for the use of the information contained in this book.

All rights reserved.
No part of this publication may be reproduced, transmitted, or stored in a retrieval system, in any form or by any means, electronic, mechanical, photocopying, recording or otherwise, without the prior permission of the publisher.

ISBN: 978–93-5304-075-8

First impression 2018

10 9 8 7 6 5 4 3 2 1

The moral right of the author has been asserted.

Printed by Parksons Graphics Pvt.Ltd., Mumbai.

This book is sold subject to the condition that it shall not, by way of trade or otherwise, be lent, resold, hired out, or otherwise circulated, without the publisher's prior consent, in any form of binding or cover other than that in which it is published.

To my son Utsav and daughter Vidushi

Contents

Introduction: Anyone Can Be Fit | ix

1: Your Career Demands Fitness | 1
2: A Mental Game | 11
3: Early Quitter Syndrome | 22
4: Eat Right, Eat Sufficient and Eat Everything | 32

SPECIAL SECTION #1: Fitness and Diet | 46

5: Fitness through Gym | 62

SPECIAL SECTION #2: Fitness through Running | 102

SPECIAL SECTION #3: Fitness through Yoga | 116

6: Style, Skin, Hygiene and Height: Fitness Enhances It All | 126

SPECIAL SECTION #4: Maintaining Fitness at Home and while on Travel | 151

7: Sexual, Physical and Mental Benefits | 162

SPECIAL SECTION #5: Fitness Tips for Women | 183

8: Exercise and Its Relationship with Injuries, Sickness and Jet Lag | 190

SPECIAL SECTION #6: Maintaining Fitness in the Office | 201

9: Second Quitter Syndrome | 208
10: Make Fitness Your Lifestyle | 223

Acknowledgments | 227

Introduction: Anyone Can Be Fit

We always ensure that our gadgets and vehicles are up to date and in fine working condition. Any small disruption and our lives go for a toss. However, when it comes to taking care of our body, we become lethargic. Why is this so? This is because when our vehicles or gadgets go kaput, they cause immediate disruptions in our routine, but our health does not deteriorate suddenly. We adjust to this gradual deterioration without realizing the danger mark. In addition, in this era of fast-paced technology promising to deliver everything at our doorsteps makes us lazy. Everything is just a click away and it hardly requires any physical activity. A new set of diseases, which used to occur rarely has now become more prevalent and is affecting a larger percentage of the population. These are lifestyle diseases, such as heart disease and diabetes, which are no longer restricted to any specific age group or rich nations. According to the report '11 Lifestyle Diseases You Should Take Seriously' published in indiatimes.com in September 2012, 'Globally 14.2 million people between the ages of 30–69 years die prematurely each year from these diseases. These diseases have emerged as bigger killers than infectious or hereditary ones. Risk factors for these diseases include tobacco use, unhealthy diets and physical inactivity.' It further details some of the diseases:

Obesity: Unhealthy eating habits and reduced physical exercise—all translate to obesity. A person with excessive weight suffers with breathing problems, blood pressure issues, cardiovascular diseases, diabetes, etc. The recent National Family Health Survey (NFHS) suggests that India currently ranks second with 155 million obese citizens and are increasing at 33–51 per cent every year.

Type II Diabetes: Obesity becomes the cause for other health problems such as Type II Diabetes which is the non-insulin dependent form, and generally develops in adults. The International Diabetes Federation (IDF) suggests that India has the largest number of people who suffer with Type II diabetes at around 40.9 million people.

Blood Pressure (BP): In India alone, more than 100 million people have high blood pressure.

Arteriosclerosis: Fatty plaques deposit in the arterial walls and cause blood circulation disorders, chest pains and heart attacks. It is linked with diabetes, obesity and a high BP. Around 30–40 per cent of deaths due to cardiovascular diseases happen in India in the age group of 34–64 years.

Heart Disease: India ranks No. 1 in patients with cardiac problems. Around 50 million people in India suffer from heart problems. The major factors involved in its development are smoking, diabetes and high cholesterol intake.

There are two types of health issues—Godsend (which we cannot control) and man-made (which we can control). We don't pay much attention to the initial symptoms, and only act when it aggravates and a medical intervention is required. We believe more in the cure than in prevention. Some even shrug it off by saying, 'Oh! It is so common!

What's the harm in taking a pill or two?'

Whenever fitness comes to our mind, we immediately discard it as if we are not cut for it. We all have a desire to be fit, flexible and healthy, but it remains limited to those on a mission to fitness. We have such a mental block that we only cite examples of those half-hearted, impatient people who did not get any result from their fitness regimes. We quickly convince ourselves to not take the trouble when a quick result is not guaranteed.

Fitness is not about six-pack abs, but it is about keeping a good health, maintaining flexibility to bend and stretch without trouble, having strength to face the mounting workloads without experiencing fatigue or stress and maintaining the right balance between body fat and muscle.

Is Achieving Fitness Really a Difficult Task?

Achieving fitness is neither difficult nor instant. It is a gradual process of transformation.

Take my word; anyone can achieve fitness irrespective of age, sex, genetic composition or lifestyle. The level of fitness may vary from person to person, but everyone can improve their well-being from their current form.

What Is the Quick Mantra To Achieve Fitness?

There are only two mantras:

1. Some level of regular physical activity
2. Food intake according to the body's requirement

Let us look into some of the common myths and realities related to fitness:

Myth: I am obese since childhood or I have a family history of obesity. Therefore, I will not be able to reduce my weight.
Reality: This is just a mental block. Even I had one during my teens. I had begun to put on weight and assumed that my body composition had always been the same, and that I will always have a paunch. Being fit includes weight reduction, increasing endurance and muscle building. Therefore, you can burn fat irrespective of your background.

Myth: How can I achieve fitness when I am not inclined to take up any physical activity?
Reality: You can still achieve fitness by doing home chores or by some daily physical activities like walking, etc. Undertaking some kind of physical exercise is always better than doing nothing. Sections 5 and 6 of this book provide advice on various exercises, which can be done easily at home even if you have as less as 15 minutes to spare.

Myth: I am a woman and I cannot go to a gym.
Reality: This is not true. Not only can women join the gym, they can also lift weights. Women can achieve fitness just like men do. They can do similar exercises, though the repetitions and counts of such exercises may vary as per their requirements. This myth is debunked beautifully in Section 5, which deals with some of the tips especially meant for women.

Myth: My job requires me to travel a lot, so I am unable to follow any fitness regimen.
Reality: You have to maintain some physical activity—either by going to a gym at the hotel or by brisk walking—whenever time permits between travels. Keeping a tab on what and when you eat is equally important, and it is better to eat moderately than to binge just because it is for free. Section

1 in this book deals with this topic.

Myth: I am differently abled, and achieving fitness will be a herculean task.
Reality: A woman in my gym is differently abled, but she is very regular and does certain exercises suitable to her ability. She is fitter compared to many others who just come to the gym, look around, try for a few weeks and then quit without any result.

Myth: Gym is boring, so I stopped going there.
Reality: Chapter 9 talks about this and other causes of dropping out from gym. It also suggests ways to avoid quitting like choosing gym partners to encourage you to visit the gym and accompanying you while workouts, to changing the music to avoid being repetitive.

Myth: I have to work long hours at office, there is no time for fitness.
Reality: Long office hours are a common excuse. Office premise itself provides enough opportunity and time to do some physical activities like exercises that can be performed at your workstation itself. Certainly, you can utilize a part of the lunch hour too. One of the expert sections deals exclusively with this topic and provides many takeaways on maintaining fitness at work.

Myth: I had taken up certain physical activities, but then got injured and I did not continue.
Reality: Exercise related injuries bothered me too and I am always very careful about them. People do face such injuries but the good news is that most of them are recoverable. Chapter 8 describes prevention from such injuries and ways to deal with them.

Myth: My profession is not the one where I need to be fit, so why worry about fitness when it has no impact on my career?

Reality: Fitness is the new currency of career. Irrespective of whether you are in a profession like hospitality or fashion, fitness does go a long way in your professional life. The first chapter of this book illustrates why fitness is important for your career irrespective of the type of profession you are in.

Myth: I know my fitness level is declining, but I don't have any ailments, so why worry?

Reality: I had the same mindset. As I aged, this mindset made things worse for me. Before it could go out of control, I undertook fitness seriously. So, don't be complacent with the current situation as prevention is always better than cure.

Myth: I tried some workouts in the past, but it has not yielded any result, so what is the guarantee that it will help me in future?

Reality: I also tried many things in the past, but never achieved satisfactory results. Now reflecting on them, actually, I never did them the right way. Doing things the right way will definitely bring positive results.

Mother of all Myths: I love food and I cannot give up anything.

Reality: Each one of us loves food. Chapter 4 and one of the expert sections talk about eating right. Isn't it that we have to be fit to enjoy the food? Eat according to what your body needs, which in turn is based on your level of physical activity. I did not give up on any particular food, but started taking it in the right quantity.

In my childhood, I spent my evenings playing games with

my friends. I was so lean and thin that my mother would always worry about my weight. I vividly remember that when I went back to school after the 10th grade summer vacation, my batch mates made fun of me for putting on weight. I now recollect that it was due to the board exams drawing near, which made me sedentary. To make things worse, my parents constantly pushed me to eat more.

The next time I put on weight was when I joined engineering college. In the initial days when one of the seniors picked me up from the hostel along with a few other freshers for a 'friendly chat', he commented that it was not good to have a paunch at that age. As sessions picked up, I began to lose weight because I had to walk from one building to another to attend classes. Once I started working, weight began to show again.

In the initial years, where walking to the bus stop to catch a bus to work did provide some exercise, as the years passed by and I graduated from bus to a more convenient mode of transportation, combined with long hours at office, my paunch started to swell again. I never thought about controlling my diet to match with my reduced physical activity.

I started brisk walking and it helped me keep things in some control. About fifteen years back, I got myself registered in a gym and must have attended it for a couple of months. I had given up soon, as I could not see any improvement. I spent more time brisk walking to compensate for the loss of hope at the gym. During that period, binging on food never stopped. About a decade ago, I consulted a dietician, and went on a diet programme. I did lose a few kilos and felt good, but continuing such a strict diet was not a practical thing to do, and soon I was back to square one.

I tried everything just like everyone else, and still got no result. With the progress of age, reduced physical activities, more responsibilities at work and feasting on tasty food, my waistline swelled to 38". I was on the borderline of being declared obese. My body fat percentage touched 30.

I realized in my mid-40s that I should take serious control over my health and since then there has been no looking back. By reclaiming fitness, I have achieved what even many folks in their 20s or 30s do not achieve.

This book is written part autobiographical with takeaways required for fitness applicable to all professionals irrespective of the background, type of job and time constraint. In addition, six fitness experts have added wider perspectives to this book to provide a holistic understanding to the readers.

I achieved fitness by hitting the gym, but the special sections in this book will also take you through other mediums like yoga, marathon, etc. for getting there. This book will answer why fitness is important and how to achieve it.

Chapter 1 talks about how fitness is becoming important for one's career in the times of increased longevity and fast changing technology, which is transforming the world and making us more sedentary.

Chapter 2 discusses the importance of having a firm determination in considering fitness as one of your life goals. It is a big leap in your journey of fitness.

Chapter 3 elaborates why so many people quit their fitness regimen in a few months of undertaking this journey.

Chapter 4 emphasizes on food and how to eat everything

but in moderate quantities, and how to control and, at the same time, enjoy the so called 'fast food', if taken wisely.

Chapter 5 talks about exercises that could be done at the gym. Even those who indulge in any kind of sports, marathons or yoga can spend a few hours in a week at the gym too. Even some hotels and offices have gyms. There are also takeaways in this chapter for non-gym goers.

Chapter 6 emphasizes on the effect of fitness on your style, skin, hygiene and height, and how it enhances your personality.

Chapter 7 discusses benefits of fitness on your sexual, mental and physical health. This chapter will show the vast benefits of fitness.

Chapter 8 focuses on injuries related with exercises and ways to prevent them.

Chapter 9 talks about ways to avoid quitting a fitness regimen when you have achieved your goal, and what happens when you quit at this stage. It also shows how to start later from where you left.

Chapter 10 emphasizes on making fitness a part of your lifestyle, your daily routine to enjoy a long and blessed life.

I have had an extensive career spanning across three decades and have been involved in many activities like angel investing, writing, learning about culture and history by criss-crossing the world. People did appreciate my efforts for my varied interests, but their actual admiration was evident when they saw me transforming into a fitter self. Seeing their enthusiasm, I started a gym in the office and initiated fitness classes like yoga and Zumba. The more difficult task was to maintain employees' initial enthusiasm towards fitness. I introduced an annual fitness competition in my organization to overcome it.

Anyone can certainly be fit. Read on and start to commit yourself to FITNESS.

ONE

Your Career Demands Fitness

The importance of health is very well understood in general, but people get puzzled when it comes to career. How can fitness help in your career? Doesn't your career depend upon your skills? It turns out that your career benefits from both. You would not want illness to act as a hindrance, especially when you have years to spend actively. There are numerous things on which you can shift the blame on—office politics, biases, discrimination—but most of the time it is you who is to be held responsible.

Here is why fitness is a necessity, not an option for your career.

Does Being Attractive Help Score Brownie Points?

I had come across a quote that said, 'This world is ruled by beautiful men and women.' While the context of this line is a far distant memory, these words lived on in my mind. Very few people are blessed with natural beauty. It is the personality that enhances beauty. Anyone can have a better personality through fitness. Not only does fitness enhance personality, it also boosts self-confidence and self-esteem.

Consider two candidates vying for a promotion or a new

job. In the hypothetical sense, if all else is the same between the two, will the more attractive person be favoured? People would jump to say 'no', because it is politically correct. However, in reality the answer is 'yes'.

Melissa Stanger in October 2012, wrote an article 'Attractive People are Simply More Successful' in www.businessinsider.com. She mentions that, 'Studies have shown that attractive people are usually hired sooner, get promotions more quickly, and are paid more than their less-attractive coworkers.' She quotes Daniel Hamermesh, who is professor of economics at the University of Texas at Austin and the author of the book *Beauty Pays: Why Attractive People Are More Successful*. According to Hamermesh, attractive people earn an average of three or four per cent more than those who are less attractive.

Unbelievable, I know, but am I right? Let's reanalyse our two-candidate scenario. Imagine you are sitting in an interview panel and a candidate walks in. The first thing you notice is the physical appearance that can create a long-lasting first impression. Attractive people always end up making an excellent first impression even before the actual conversation begins. It does not mean that skills, qualification or suitability of the role becomes secondary; it simply means that first impression reflects your personality.

The same article further quotes another article from *Psychology Today* by Dario Maestripieri, a professor of comparative human development, evolutionary biology and neurobiology at the University of Chicago saying that 'Beautiful people tend to bring in more money for their companies, and are therefore seen as more valuable employees and harder workers. A door-to-door insurance salesman is better able to sell to customers who find him attractive.'

Now, we all agree that there are some professions where personality matters the most. The hospitality and fashion industry are prime examples. However, you might ask, 'Why should we worry about fitness when most jobs do not have such requirements or expectations?' Let me explain. It is true that most jobs don't place lofty expectations on employees' fitness, but it will not be right to confine fitness to only those in specific industries. Confused?

Hamermesh, in the same article, says, 'Beauty may just reflect self-esteem. Perhaps people's self-confidence manifests itself in their behaviour, so that their looks are rated more highly, and their self-esteem makes them more desirable and higher-paid employees.' 'Another possibility is that beauty and the attractiveness of one's personality are positively related, and that it is the general sparkle of one's personality, not one's beauty, that increases earnings,' he adds.

Now, it should be clear that irrespective of the type of profession, such desirable personality traits do have varying degree of appeal to employers.

What can you do if you don't consider yourself attractive? You cannot change the way you look or your height. What you can certainly change is your overall personality through fitness. So, first take solace that anyone can become attractive and that too at any stage of their life.

Thus, get rid of this self-doubt and don't hope to scurry away into a job that doesn't seem to require physical fitness. No matter what your profession is, it will require a level of fitness. The lack of it can hamper your job prospects and career growth. Certainly, the level and type of fitness and its impact on the job varies from profession to profession. Some professions like modelling are short-lived if fitness is not maintained from the beginning.

Do Organizations Realize That Fitness Increases Productivity?

In this millennium, organizations have been focusing more on fitness. They have been opening gyms or providing gym memberships if they do not have one; and conducting fitness classes like yoga, Zumba and Aerobics, and even encouraging activities like trekking, cycling and marathon running through sponsorship.

So why are they doing this? Is this true altruism or do these organizations get something in return?

Ron Friedman's article 'Regular Exercise is Part of Your Job,' published in the *Harvard Business Review*, suggests that exercising during regular office hours may enhance your performance. It cites the result of a Leeds Metropolitan University study, which examined the influence of daytime exercise among office workers with access to a company gym. In the study, researchers had over 200 employees self-report their performance on a daily basis. Then, they examined fluctuations amongst employees by comparing their output on days when they exercised to those when they did not. They reported that they were able to manage their time more effectively; they were more productive and had smoother interactions with their colleagues. They went home more satisfied.

The same Leeds Metropolitan University study is cited in another interesting article 'Positive Effects of Exercise on Work Performance' by Dan Ketchum, published in healthyliving.azcentral.com. It raises a question that exercise releases a chemical in the brain. Positive effects of exercise on your personal life also influence your workplace. It says:

> Work performance increases because in addition to sharpening mental performance, regular physical activity

improves time-management skills, which in turn improve your ability to meet deadlines. Business owners who offer company exercise programs find that on-site exercise decreases turnaround time. Exercise causes an overall work performance boost of about 15 per cent, according to a 2005 study performed by health professor Jim McKenna of Leeds Metropolitan University. Harvard researchers find that post-workout blood flow creates the optimal conditions for performing tasks that require focused thinking.

Employees build organizations; so fitter the employees, the better will be the organization.

Are We Worshipping Young Achievers or Supporting Age-based Discrimination?

In this millennium, we are praising young achievers. The headlines are beaming with 'Company xyz has got her youngest CEO at the age of 32', 'Here are powerful people under 30', 'Successful habits of young and fast achievers', 'Life lessons from young Turks and how they built their ventures', and so on.

Despite our best efforts to try to be one of them, most of us do not fall in this category. One must keep pursuing what we desire or dream of, but it is also true that with each day passing, we are growing older. As time slips by, it gets more difficult to fit into the same workspace filled with younger and fitter co-workers. In addition, it gets worse when you have to work *for* these youngsters sitting at higher or more influential positions.

What is your initial reaction?

You convince yourself that you have a plethora of

experience and your employer cannot overlook it, but clocking up years in the job might not be fruitful. The skills acquired in the past might not be fully relevant in current circumstances unless it can be abstracted to apply in the newer areas. Traditional jobs are being replaced with new ones. So, without upgrading your skills your experience means nothing. However, one should not ignore soft skills like work ethics, discipline, punctuality, patience under crisis and many others, which will never be outdated. The movie *The Intern* is a classic example of how a 70-year-old retired man took advantage of his experience to get a job.

However, the question arises—do companies discriminate based on age? Certainly not, as every company has a written policy against it and any violation is penalized. However, is the implementation of this policy firm?

No! Let us come back to the previous situation about the candidate who came for an interview. After the first impression, the next thing an interviewer notices is the body language and then self-confidence. Many subtleties help to create an overall impression that can make or break your prospects. Candidates labelled as 'senior', 'very experienced' and 'over qualified' are rejected in the first go. The typical responses for rejecting such candidates are:

> 'The person lacks the enthusiasm towards this new challenging and highly visible job.'
> 'This job has a lot of travelling and the candidate appears to lack energy.'
> 'He has all the required skills, but it is doubtful if he will be able to gel with the rest of the team which has less experience and so would prefer someone who's good with teamwork.'

These candidates don't seem to be 'fit' for the job. The word 'fit' is used for 'suitability' here. Nevertheless, these comments can be reversed if you are 'physically fit' and exhibit confidence, positive energy and positive attitude. After all, age is just a number, not a state of being.

Eventually, your physical age will begin to matter less as your fitness will steal the spotlight and the chances of your acceptability will increase manifold.

Is Work-related Stress Hurting Career Growth?

Everyone says that his or her work is stressful. Some do it to brag about how busy they are or to show off their self-importance, while others genuinely mean it. Stress, however, is an individualistic matter. A person equipped with better subject matter and time management skills can execute the same amount of work within a stipulated amount of time with lesser stress. The amount of stress one can handle is vital for his or her career. Here, fitness comes handy, as many scientific reports suggest that fitness could help in reducing stress. This will help in managing current responsibilities in a better way. Imagine if you are unable to handle your current workload, it is natural for your management to not be willing to consider you for bigger responsibilities.

Can Fitness Help Stay Afloat during Unemployment?

We are bombarded daily with news about lay-offs and shutdowns leading to loss of jobs. What is the connection between fitness and losing jobs? Can we really say that fit people are less likely to be laid off?

Not really! If a company decides to close down a product line, a division or exits from a certain business, it will not matter how fit or skilled you are. You will find yourself without a job anyway. However, fitness can help you during this layoff period.

According to an article in expertrain.com, 'How Fitness Can Help You Survive Unemployment', author Paula Beaton mentions,

> Unemployment can lead to anxiety, depression, low self-esteem and even weight gain. Without your job to motivate you, it can be hard to find the energy to workout at the gym or go for a run. Even your social life and personal relationships can suffer. But fitness can actually help you banish those unemployment blues—you'll boost your self-confidence, build endurance and strength and increase your energy levels, which could make job hunting less stressful.

If you lose your job, you are likely to face some of the below-mentioned issues.

Doubts about self-worth: When you lose a job, your self-confidence and sense of self-worth will take a hit. When your spirits and self-esteem are low, finding a new job will be even more difficult. Life is made up of many other things apart from work. Having a hobby—good fitness regime, supportive family and a social circle—plays an important role in living a holistic life.

Lack of focus: You may feel disillusioned. You could also experience lack of concentration, which is necessary to develop new skills, undertake training, pursue education or even focus on searching a job. A regular workout schedule will help you bring back your ability to focus, as all exercises require concentration and attention to specific body parts.

Sloppy daily schedule: You are used to a daily schedule when you have a job. However, there is no need to adhere to any schedule in an out of job scenario. When your daily schedule goes haywire, it triggers other challenges too. Fitness routine can enforce regularity, which induces a balanced mood and encourages a more systematic job search.

Need for a network: What do you need when you lose a job? A network. A gym can be a great place for networking. One day at my gym, a man hopped onto the treadmill next to mine and started a conversation with me. After a few weeks of occasional meetings, he asked me my name and where I worked. Initially, I was reluctant to share, but relented. A few weeks later, he approached me and said, 'I googled you and now I want some career advice from you!'

He followed up by sending me his curriculum vitae. I suggested some leads and he followed up with them. He found himself a new job soon.

There are many other benefits too which a gym provides during unemployment. I have met a few of them, who have found happiness or satisfaction at the gym as it gave them a sense of achieving something and that not everything was lost.

Those who equate a life to their job face a grave problem during such periods, but people with hobbies and a fitness regime certainly have a higher chance of bouncing back. So, do not give up hope and continue the fitness regime. This will help you while you are unemployed, as exercising is a stress reliever and situations like this might become stressful.

Is Fitness the New Weapon against Current Career Challenges?

In the last chapter of my previous book *Faster Smarter*

Higher: Managing Your Career, I dealt with three realities of today:

1. Increased life expectancy.
2. An organization's inability to provide job security and its employees' inability to pledge their loyalty towards the organization.
3. With fluctuations in companies' stakes on a quarterly or yearly basis, unpredictability is forcing people to prepare for some kind of cushion for future job losses by trying to earn more in lesser time.

Like a typical product cycle, your career also has four stages: Introduction, growth, maturity and decline. Organizations try to add more features to their products to ensure its relevance and extend its maturity. Similarly, you need to refine and acquire skills that help you stay relevant and delay your career's decline. This decline, however, is inevitable. Therefore, as organizations launch new products before the decline of the previous one, you must also start reinventing yourselves in advance to extend your shelf life.

I believe that fitness is the foundation required to fulfil the above suggestions. A good fitness regime can help you maintain your health—a key ingredient in extending your career. I am experiencing the benefits of this newfound youthfulness and energy as I enter the fourth decade of my career.

Just imagine how long you can take care of your career if you cannot take care of yourself.

This fitness is not an option but a necessity for you, your career and for all others to whom you matter.

TWO

A Mental Game

On a Monday morning back in November 2011, one of my colleagues told me that when he was trying on clothes, he looked into the mirror and realized that he was totally out of shape.

I had been experiencing the same sentiments for several years now. I added that even my triglyceride levels had crossed their limits a few years ago and that my cholesterol level was reaching the upper limit. He mentioned that he was thinking of joining a gym. I always associated the word 'gym' with injuries and lack of effectiveness, as I had never seen any change in the people who claimed to go to the gym or used fitness equipment at home. I spoke to him about my dilemmas associated with gyms. He told me that one should at least give it a chance. For years, my workout used to be 20 minutes of brisk walking and I, somehow, managed to keep my waist size at 36". Gradually, I could see that despite increasing my brisk walking to 35 minutes, my waist size had increased to 38" and remained at that. A couple of days ago while getting ready for a party, my wife commented on how unfit I had become and asked me if I would have the will power to reduce my weight. So, when my colleague suggested joining a gym, I decided to give it a shot. My diet programmes from the past certainly helped me reduce some weight, but I could not stick to it long. After all, the lure of sweets and junk food is hard to resist.

That evening I told to my wife that I was going to join a gym. She did not question the sincerity of my decision. She only wondered how long it would take me to give up, considering I had never played any kind of sport in my life. It was good that she did not voice her thoughts, instead encouraged me to look for a gym.

> **Tip!** Entering a fitness regime is a mental game. Just as in any other game, the more you practice the right way, the more you gain; fitness is no different. The more you do a systematic investment in it, better will be the result.

I realized later that determination is a key to fitness. First, you should make up your mind that you must be fit. You can have many options to achieve it—playing sports, joining the gym, aerobics or Zumba, yoga and so on.

> **Caution:** Most of the time, people come for quick gain, which hardly provides any result. They quickly form an opinion that their fitness regime is not helping them, losing the opportunity to enjoy the fitness.

My office did not have a gym at that time. So, my first concern was whether I should choose a gym near my office or home. I preferred the latter, as it would be accessible over weekends. If you have a gym at office and/or at your residential complex, it makes things easy, but you still have to evaluate the various criteria mentioned below to find a suitable gym.

As far as fitness is concerned, it matters little whether the gym is high class or average. What really matters is the type and spread of equipment and how they are maintained. One must also consider the hygiene of changing rooms and shower facilities. Besides, not only the experience of trainers but also their success rate with their clients are very important.

The second most important criterion is the location of the gym. It should be easily accessible either from home or office or both.

> **Tip!** The fitness center should have sufficient well-maintained facilities and its location should be such that when you pass by it, you should get a tinge of guilt for skipping it.

I went to a nearby gym and met the person in charge. I signed up with the gym for three months to start with, but people can start with anything from a month to a year. My decision to take up a three-month membership was purely a mental block—whether I would be able to workout at this age or not.

When I went to the gym the other day, I also enquired about their personal trainers, especially the ones who had helped sedentary people belonging to my age group in the past. He mentioned two names—one from the morning and the other from the evening session. I chose evening timings as I leave for work early in the morning. He then gave a call to the trainer to inform him about a prospective client.

Suddenly, while talking to him, the gym in charge sized

me up and said, 'OK, OK type' on the phone. I could not resist smiling, as I was sure that the trainer was asking about my condition to decide upon how much effort will be required. I asked the in charge about my assumption and he embarrassingly confirmed the same. I signed up for a month's session with the personal trainer with an understanding that if I get positive results, I will extend it.

> **Tip!** Getting the right trainer or coach is a very important milestone in your journey towards fitness. As commercialization is seeping in, personal trainers do not give full attention to their trainees as they are constantly on the lookout for more clients. You should discuss this before signing up.

There is no dearth of fitness facilities, but there is a dearth of sincerity in trainers or coaches. It is also advisable to not give them an idea that you are signing up for a short duration as their focus on you will also be limited for that period only. Therefore, they will not be able to get you on to the right track for holistic benefits. If you have an understanding with them that you are eager to continue based on the progress, it will motivate them to go an extra mile to help you. Certainly, the decision to continue will always be the client's prerogative.

Many a times, people cannot afford the trainer or don't want to spend on them as they are not fully convinced that they need one. In such situations, it is important to have a 'buddy' or a partner. A buddy can be your friend, colleague or a member of your fitness facility. Your buddy must be a couple of notches above you and passionate about fitness. He or she should have a good and extensive experience to guide and motivate you and should be able to drag you to the facility when you feel lazy.

However, working out with friends can be counterproductive too. Most of the time, a bunch of friends decide to hit a gym. I have noticed that they come around the same time, talk a lot and check their phones continuously, use a few weights, tease each other, do some treadmills and look into the mirror to size up their arms and abs. If you are joining a gym or any other fitness activity with your friends, it is important that motivation to attend will run high, so that even if one or two drop out, someone will certainly accompany you. However, with the passage of time some of the friends will drop out citing various reasons. These could be lack of time, no progress and change in work timings among other things. Some go to the extremes and decide to drop out when they don't make any progress compared to their friends. Such situations will demotivate you to proceed with your fitness plan.

All the above will help you in taking the right steps so that you can adhere to the fitness regime. I have seen people who are mentally quite firm in the beginning, but do not follow the above-mentioned suggestions; even their strong will power does not last long.

Another very common trick is bonding around a common hobby. For determination, it is also important to bond with people that will also expand your circle of friends and you will learn a lot too. Even downloading an app in your phone around your hobby will boost your determination. But why should a stranger become your buddy?

You respond to someone when they ask you something. If you begin to like the interaction, you will be more forthcoming to share information. Some of them might not be willing to interact a lot, but you will certainly find some who are more forthcoming. So, try to reach out to a couple of fitness freaks who are at an advance level and seem trustworthy. Make that person your buddy, exchange phone numbers, synchronize your timings and leverage the experience.

Despite all the above suggestions, there will be days or times when you will not have a personal trainer or a buddy. In such days, you should not hesitate to seek help from other trainers or coaches at the fitness facility. Ask multiple times if things are unclear. You can also take their support while exercising. Your fitness is important and they are there to help you. Do not be shy. Such type of help will be required in the initial months. When I was signing up with my personal trainer, I remember my gym in charge telling me that every trainer has his or her own strengths. He asked me to tell my trainer to seek inputs from other trainers in guiding me if the results are not as per expectations. This was a very useful advice, which I realized later and followed it.

> **Caution** Fitness is a very wide subject and no single trainer, coach or buddy will be able to guide you throughout the journey. It is common to change them as per need or with time. When you hit the plateau, you should seek inputs from videos, talk to other members and trainers and come out with a new plan.

However, there are many who don't sign up for a personal trainer, coach or reach out to a buddy. The reasons could be many. Not being able to find the right trainer who can understand your needs and guide you accordingly could be one of the many reasons. The timing of the trainer or buddy may not match. Sometimes the trainer's knowledge is limited and is still learning on the job. At times, his attitude becomes a problem. It could be anything; therefore, videos and articles, which are free of cost and easily available on the Internet, come to the rescue. Some of these videos are quite good and informative. However, as they are not a substitute for a real person in the gym, it will be helpful to keep a few things in mind. You should exercise in a certain manner—right posture, with the correct breathing practice, a mental focus on what body part you are targeting, and how long should you wait between the repetitions for the routine to be effective. If you can get these right, you can do them on your own. Such plethora of information on the internet should be first carefully skimmed for veracity of truth and then can be used to weigh the options suggested in the gym. Sometimes, I too have discussed such information with a few members and trainers of the gym to choose the right one in each situation.

Next day, I went to the gym and met my trainer. He was young, energetic and enthusiastic. For a moment, I wondered how much experience he would have to help me in this journey, but his soft skills were quite good and he immediately made me comfortable. First, we exchanged our phone numbers, and he made a sharp comment with a smile: 'I will be troubling you to make sure that you are regular. If you are so, you will definitely see the result. Leave the rest on me.'

His self-confidence was quite reassuring. He introduced me to the gym physiotherapist and I underwent a full-body checkup. She noted the measurements of various parts of my body using different types of scales. Some of the data were mentioned in a file, and the rest were entered into a computer for the record. The measurements also included my initial body fat, lean body mass, Body Mass Index (BMI) and many other factors. My body fat was around 30 per cent. The google search revealed how far I was from the ideal body fat percentage for my age and I was happy to have joined the gym.

I had to undertake a treadmill test to get the threshold heart beat to determine safe and effective level for cardio exercise. This is important to avoid any injuries and health related issues as people usually begin with running on the treadmill, lifting weights for longer durations without knowing their pre- and post-exercises and threshold heart rate. A complete body check-up provides a safe range to run or walk on the treadmill. Now, majority of wristwatches or bands are fitted with heart rate sensors for self-monitoring.

The details of all the tests with suggestions were handed over to my trainer. Such tests by the gym were conducted at regular intervals to measure the progress and accordingly alter the exercises.

> **Caution** Skipping the health checks to ascertain the level of cardiovascular exercises and the pre- and post-exercises will neither be beneficial nor will they provide the desired result. This will lead to a feeling of waste of time.

Initially, my trainer said that I would be doing a lot of cardio vascular exercises followed with some floor exercises to slowly loosen the muscle. I was told that I could use weights later. In the gym, I observed people at various fitness levels and I wondered how they had reached the stages. My trainer used to narrate success stories of people and the way they had transformed themselves. He also mentioned that some people have been regulars for years, but have not changed, as their exercises were sub optimal. He reminded me that if I were regular, he would bring gradual changes in me.

The first day went well. I came back home feeling happy that I was now a gym goer. I was expecting to get some appreciation from my spouse, but nothing came my way.

Next day, I proudly announced to as many people as possible in the office that I had joined the gym. Some smiled, others were curious to see how long I would continue. They smirked as they had seen many people making such bold statements. No one took me seriously; neither did they laugh at me nor discourage me.

> **Tip!** Make your fitness routine public to maintain the pressure of continuing this journey.

That afternoon, I was in a meeting, when my phone rang and it was my trainer. For a moment, I thought that on the very second day, he was planning to take off or come late. I was getting angry and excused myself to take the call. 'Sorry for the call, sir, but please do come. I will be waiting for you. Even if you are busy or late, please feel free to text me, but don't skip.' It seemed like he was used to such excuses. He sounded reassured when I told him that I would be going to the gym.

My schedule started with a mix of treadmill, cycling and cross training, which he chose in a combination for cardiovascular exercises. He stood next to me all the time to ensure that I do not reduce the speed. Once completed, he made me do some more stretches and light floor exercises.

A few days later, he introduced me to weights. I was happy that finally even I will get to use dumbbells. I thought of asking him to take a picture of me with the dumbbells to post it on social media. He asked me to pick a dumbbell of a comfortable size. I went ahead and then picked the one that weighed 3 kgs. He came closer and looked at me puzzled.

'Sir, these are good for girls. You should have picked a heavier one.'

I would have blasted him as my anger was brewing. Nevertheless, I controlled myself when I noticed that he said it out of concern and on a rather serious note.

'Let me first go ahead with these,' I replied.

'OK, then you will have to do more repetitions,' he added.

These dumbbells were comfortable for me, but as the counts started to increase, it became more difficult and he began to help me in completing few of the last counts.

He allowed me to take a short break and repeated the second set and later, the third too, where I needed more help from him.

My anger quickly evaporated and so did my dream of posting the picture.

'Sir, the 3-kg weights were difficult for you. You were right to begin with them,' he said with a smile.

'When can I move to 5 kgs?' I asked impatiently.

'If you continue doing the exercises with me regularly, you will soon move on to the 5-kg weights. When doing the exercise, make sure that you focus on that body part that is being exercised. This will help you,' he replied.

> **Tip!** Being regular in the chosen fitness activity and doing the right exercises in a right way is a step forward towards fitness.

It is truly a mental game. Determination is a key to sustain the initial enthusiasm in this beautiful journey called fitness. I continued in this journey mostly due to the dreams, which were sold to me by my trainer and I bought them, building more on them. This cycle has basically helped me to set a step-by-step goal towards achieving fitness in a new unchartered world. It just needs your determination to overcome a roller-coaster ride in this journey, as you will witness in the upcoming chapters.

THREE

Early Quitter Syndrome

Two weeks had passed doing basic exercises. So far, my determination was holding on. I could see that other members in the gym had their tees drenched in sweat, whereas mine would be largely dry. I was determined to change that gradually, but my progress was quite slow. I was more careful about any exercise, which could have adversely affected my knee and spine. I was somewhat paranoid about it and bugged my trainer so much that when he tried to take me to the next level, he was very cautious. At my age, quick goals are not possible, so I had to be content with this slow speed. I could see that a few serious new members, younger in age, who joined around the same time as me, were moving to the next level faster than I was.

My gym is a happening place as it is close to a college and a few offices. This helps to draw a younger set of people to try their hands on fitness. Many stories are told here, which seem amusing to the onlookers. There are a few members who are loud, demanding, those who show-off, and then there are some who are self-obsessed and hate to share equipment. It was December and the number of gym-goers were growing, and people had to wait for their turn to use the equipment. I was getting a little frustrated. I was pressed for time, and I needed to get on to those machines quickly to keep the break between my exercises to the least. My trainer used to calm me down by teaching me alternative exercises whenever any equipment was busy.

'Why is the gym so crowded suddenly? It would be difficult for me to get the desired result if I am unable to use the equipment,' I vented to my trainer.

'This is a temporary phase; it happens every year, sir,' he replied.

I looked at him inquisitively.

'They want to get in shape before the New Year's party. Then in January, some more will come to accomplish their New Year's resolutions. Later, some more will come to get ready for Valentine's Day. All of them would want quick results and this rush will die out by mid-February.' He smiled as he explained.

'We are happy to get the membership fees, but such shortcut approach will hardly be of any use,' he continued.

> **Tip!** You can set two types of intermediate goals. First, occasion-based goals (e.g., to be fit for a New Year's party) are those where you have to work backwards and join the fitness facility much before the event, not just a few weeks. Second, milestone-based goals (like losing 5 kgs) are those where you have to make a humble beginning and remain persistent to achieve the result.

'So why don't they continue once they join the gym?' I asked.

'Sir, they are not serious about their intentions to begin the training. They just want to get a temporary fix for a particular occasion. Most of them fail or a few achieve partial success. Irrespective of the result, they feel that they have done a good job.' He spoke like a wise man.

I did not want to challenge his opinions, as I wanted him to continue with the daily entertainment.

'Do you know that guy?' he pointed at an overweight person.

'He joined the gym last year. He was way overweight. I managed to reduce his weight by 10 kgs. He was happy. He got engaged and stopped coming to the gym. He again went back to where he had started.'

I looked at him in astonishment.

'The girl called off the engagement due to his obesity. That was when he rejoined gym.'

'So sad!' I exclaimed.

It is appalling that we don't have any regard for others' privacy, but that is how our society is and my trainer is no different.

'But then this is not good. He should have persisted with his weight-loss goals,' I continued.

'Exactly, sir. But no one adheres to such suggestions.'

Such knee-jerk approach towards fitness does not do any good other than a few great pictures. Early quitters should be cognizant of this fact.

> **Caution** If you undertake fitness activities with an intention to quit soon, it will do you more harm than good. Fitness is not a punishment; it is a requirement for a healthy living.

One day while doing floor exercises, I was lying on my back. My trainer bent both of my legs pushed them slowly towards my chest, and in the end, he gave another sudden push to complete the stretch before straightening them out. That push triggered a severe pain in the muscles around my ribs, as if my bone and muscles got separated from each other. The severity of the pain made him nervous and he immediately straightened me up and told me to relax. He began to apologize profusely. The pain reduced slowly, but it was still there. A few exercises were still remaining, but he let me go home after a few relaxing exercises. I braced myself for some painful weeks. My wife gave me an ice pack to apply on the bruise and suggested to contact our general physician. Luckily, I got an appointment for the next morning. I took some painkillers to survive the night. On hearing that I had joined a gym, my doctor smiled and asked about my entire exercise routine. He did a full-body check-up and said that whatever my trainer told me to do was right. He assured that it would slowly heal. He gave me some medicines to reduce the muscle pain and told me to take it for two weeks. He also told me to have calcium, protein, vitamin D and vitamin B12 in adequate quantities during a fitness regime. He also mentioned that an overdose or underdose of these could be harmful.

> **Tip!** Irrespective of age, a periodic consultation with a doctor is important during any fitness regime. It will ensure that you are not injuring any part of your body unknowingly.

After hearing from my doctor that my trainer was on the right track, my anger somewhat subsided. That day, I reached office a bit late and had a lot of pending work to clear, and before I could realize, it was already late afternoon. My phone rang.

'Hello, sir! How is your pain?' My trainer was on the

other side. There was no remorse in his tone, which made me angry again.

'A little better. My doctor has prescribed some medicines for the pain.' I deliberately hid the fact that he was following the right exercise routine.

'Good, sir! I am very happy that you are taking medicines. Please do come today. We will focus on your lower body, so that the upper body can rest. Don't skip just because of the pain.'

My trainer, who must be almost half my age, had taken full responsibility of me and, in a way, was telling me to obey his orders. My anger dissipated immediately seeing the earnest sincerity in his tone and I agreed to go to the gym.

> **Caution** Do not quit due to early signs of pain or discomfort. Instead, share your doctor's advice with your trainer or buddy who can fine-tune the exercise.

While doing my lower body exercises, I noticed a new member who was quite tall and thin. However, his biceps were bulging and they were disproportionately larger than the rest of his body. He appeared like a tall palm tree with two coconuts hanging from his shoulders. I was puzzled, so I enquired about the exercises he was doing. My trainer smiled and said that the trainee was under a transformation stage. My curiosity did not die there; my trainer explained that he used to be very thin and had recently started taking protein supplements to bulk-up.

'How did you know this?' I asked enquiringly.

'We are in this profession and know that for faster results some people take protein supplements.'

'So, for faster results, should you use protein supplement?' I asked.

'Not always. There are some who take supplements because they need more protein to maintain themselves. Then there are some who do not get the sufficient quantity of protein through meals, so they have to take it. Some take it immediately after the workout, as it provides faster absorption, so they use protein like whey,' he continued.

'You don't need to take it. I suggest you go natural. As said earlier, you should take sufficient protein in your diet to bulk-up naturally.'

There is no right or wrong as far as protein supplements are concerned, however, the intake quantity should depend upon your metabolism. On enquiring from my doctor, he also agreed with my trainer and suggested that I should go natural. He also suggested that those who take supplements should get their kidney creatinine level checked regularly to avoid any side effects due to overdose.

> **Caution** If you are on a very high natural protein diet, or consume protein supplements or steroids for a quick turnaround, you should regulate the dosage and consult the doctor to negate any possibilities of side effects on your kidneys or other organs.

Some of my colleagues ask me what motivated me to go to the gym, as almost a month had passed and they could not see any significant change. I too was confused, but then, it was too early for me to decide that the gym will not help me. I did not want to be a quitter, but a thought did come to my mind that my trainer was probably hiding the fact that my chances of becoming fit are bleak; nonetheless he wanted to try.

He kept citing a few success stories. I too kept asking when could I become like one of these fitter people at the gym. Initially, he avoided my questions and when I insisted, he made it clear that I will see some results only after a few months. He was gradually progressing in my case due to my body condition and repeated warnings to avoid injury at any cost. He told me that what a regular person could achieve in three months, I might take longer. He also added that it was not because he wanted to make money for a longer period, but slow and steady would certainly win the race. So long a wait, I thought to myself. When you hear stories of a quick turnaround, *long* is demotivating and the thought of quitting is natural to occur.

> **Tip!** Do not compare your progress with others'. Everybody is different; they eat differently and their exercises are different. It is advisable to focus on oneself rather than on others. Others could be used as role models to set realistic self-goals for yourself.

Slowly my pain subsided, but did not go away completely. I already extended my trainer's services to three months and he was happy and over enthusiastic.

He made me do a new leg exercise. The exercise was not difficult or painful, but after some time, I felt a pain in my leg. Slowly, I found it difficult to walk. I asked him about my condition and he said that such pains are normal, and it should go away in a couple of days. He suggested me to check on the Internet about such pains. I was getting into a foul mood. Somehow, I managed to reach home.

My wife could sense my frustration with the gym. She asked me pointedly: 'Are you a quitter?'

I would have quit had she not posed that question to me. I checked on the Internet and again the trainer was right. It said that the pain stays for a few days and then goes away, but then a few days had passed and there was no improvement. I consulted my doctor again and he reconfirmed that my trainer was doing the right exercises. Again, he gave me some medicines and told me that it would take some time to recover. It took around seven to ten days to recover completely, but then I was not allowed to rest for more than a day or two. My trainer's calls made me go to the gym. He told me that he would focus on my upper body more as my lower body was still recovering. I did not know whether to laugh or cry, but his determination and my wife's probing questions did not let me quit the gym.

Just a few months into fitness, I had seen many people quit due to various reasons other than the aforementioned ones:

Some of them cite lack of focus by the trainer or buddy. If you are feeling this, go and talk to the person about the issue. The reason could also be you. Some members take inputs but don't adhere to them and thereby the trainer or buddy loses interest. If you do not agree with your trainer's suggestions, do consult and involve them in your decisions so that you benefit from it the most.

Some people want to build muscles fast, and they go for a quick bulk-up. This process involves putting on a lot of weight hoping that with right exercises, they will be able to turn the bulk into muscles. The whole process is difficult and requires dedication, and if you lose focus at any point of time, you will not get the required benefit.

Normally, in every fitness facility, there are peak hours, which are usually mornings and evenings. If the facility does not have sufficient space to accommodate its members at a time, they have to wait long for the equipment to be free. At times, they don't even get to use them and decide to quit. However, I have seen some pair up with another member to use equipment alternatively. This is a good idea as it will also enable bonding and you might make good friends too.

Some of them also quit due to a change in their work schedule not leaving enough time. But the major reason for leaving any activity is the lack of satisfactory improvement in one's fitness. My routine continued and there were hardly any changes visible, though there was some loss of weight. I could also feel that my body was more flexible than it used to be. My trainer was alarmed when I shared my frustration with him. He advised me against leaving because those who have left the gym at this stage have hardly come back.

I was impressed by his honesty to agree that people do quit due to the lack of visible changes. I asked him what I should do to make the changes visible that would boost my confidence.

I saw him smile sheepishly for the first time.

He said, 'Sir, actually, I have not seen any of my clients continue beyond three months. So, I cannot say for sure how things will turn out for you.'

I was astonished, but he quickly added.

'You must trust me. I would want to do a few experiments on you and I am sure it will yield positive results.'

For a moment, I felt cheated and thought of changing the gym. After some time, he stopped taking payments for being my personal trainer, but continued to help and guide me as he used to.

I assured myself then that there was no guarantee that another place would be better. Sensing my dilemma, he continued, 'You have determination and as you have survived three months, you will certainly see the results.'

Being already reassured from my doctor in the past that he was doing the right exercises, I trusted him, and thus, survived the quitter syndrome. This is a major turning point in anyone's journey towards fitness.

> **Tip!** There are many reasons to quit a fitness regime. Always tell this to yourself 'I am not a quitter. I will show my determination to make a change in my life.' This attitude will help you overcome any negative feelings.

FOUR

Eat Right, Eat Sufficient and Eat Everything

The importance of food to maintain fitness is known to everyone. Some recommend extreme dos and don'ts, but as I have gone through a diet plan in the past, I know it is difficult to maintain a strict one. Food is very important in our lives. It is a major criterion for any successful ceremony. Any get together cannot be complete without discussing restaurants and their specialties. We celebrate good news with friends and food, and sometimes our outings are directed to a specific food joint or dhaba. On weekends, restaurants are full of professionals rewarding themselves after a week-long arduous work. We cannot change it; this is how we are. Food is often accompanied by free-flowing alcohol, as it provides relaxation, and most importantly, it bonds us with our friends. However, important business dinners with alcohol act in two ways—either to acquire more information about other's businesses or to break the ice in stalemate negotiations.

From day one of my fitness regime, I had decided that I will eat everything but in moderation. However, the term moderation is very loosely used. People interpret it at will and indulge in food and alcohol based on their moods or occasions, and most of the time they come up with a reason to justify. That is why dieticians tend to make some foods forbidden, as most of us lack the will power to control ourselves.

One of the main reasons why we become overweight and then obese are that we simply eat more than what our body needs. I have come across people who binge on food, and justify the excess weight with things like broader bones, heredity or a low rate of metabolism. It is not just the quantity of food, but the type and frequency as well. In addition, what matters is the daily activity that balances the intake of the food.

> **Tip!** Moderate your daily food intake. You will slowly become more aware of your body requirements.

In Special Section 1 of this book, a dietician has provided ways to overcome the obsession over food, but here are my experiences. These tips can easily be followed in a busy schedule. It is just a discipline. Some people put reminders on their mobiles, some put stickers at their workstations, while others use small breaks wisely if they are too busy.

1. **Do not to eat when hungry:** Eat small portions at regular intervals of 2–3 hours even when you don't feel like it. When we are advised to eat smaller portions of food more frequently, we tend to eat in addition to the current high intake rather than reducing the overall intake. This advice then proves to be a bogus as it triggers weight gain. To eat nominal quantities periodically is the mantra.
2. **The old saying** goes as 'breakfast like a king, lunch like a prince and dine like a pauper.' Until late afternoon, you

can eat as per your schedule and even if you have to occasionally binge on food, do so latest by late afternoon. Do not overeat in the evening. Certainly, dinner has to be very light and you must finish dinner at least two to three hours before you go to sleep. I take an early dinner and still attend late-night calls few days during the week without any issues.

> **Caution** Sitting for a late night call with beverages or snacks, affects your health adversely. Drinking water should be sufficient.

3. **Dinnertime essentials** is a bowl of salad. If you cannot avoid rice, try a few spoons only to satisfy your taste buds. You should have proteins like dal, rajma, beans or chicken. You can add one spoonful of ghee to it and have chapatti/*phulka*/roti without butter and a small portion of cooked vegetables.
4. If **feeling hungry just before sleeping**, have a cup of milk with or without jaggery, curd or buttermilk.
5. **Record your weight periodically at the same time of the day** to rule out the fluctuation in the weight, which happens throughout the day. Fluctuation of a kilogram in a day is normal. If it increases, spend more time doing cardiovascular exercises, watch your food intake and it should come down to a normal level.
6. **Water intake** should be around 3 litres per day. You can start with 2 litres as well. Drink water at regular intervals if possible, but remember to keep these intervals short. Some folks set a reminder on their laptops to take a short walk and drink water regularly. As the level of fitness increases, your water intake also increases. Water

intake quantity is also dependent upon your body weight and some other parameters.

7. **Snacking** comes with a price. Do not think that a fistful of snacks is harmless as it is just a small amount. A major cause of weight gain is this habit of snacking. So, whenever you feel hungry, eat some nuts (almonds and walnuts should be preferred, but peanuts or cashews can be fine too). However, do not eat more than a fistful of nuts in a day, yes, in a full day. After a while, if you feel hungry again, you could drink water, green/herbal tea or a healthy snack.

8. **Avoid feeling a need to snack.** There are days when you are very hungry. In addition to your normal two and a half hours intake, you get pangs to eat more. As said earlier, you can have some nuts and fruits, but not too frequently in a day. So, to kill such irregular untimely snack pangs, keep some clove or cardamom with you. Just chew a few and drink water; hunger pangs will subside soon.

9. **Office lunch blues:** Some of the companies provide lunch to their employees. You should be selective in eating only what is good for you, as most of the time the servings are quite big and often unhealthy. You should order small portions of food when you go out with colleagues. When you chat and eat, you tend to indulge more than required, and if the meal is biryani, pulao or dishes with rich gravies served with breads soaked in butter, losing weight becomes difficult even for those who exercise regularly, as it nullifies the gain. Jennifer Cohen, in her article '9 Bad Habits that Make you Fat' for *Forbes*, wrote,

If your friends or spouse overeats, you're 57 per cent more likely to overeat too, according to research from the New England Journal of Medicine. I am NOT suggesting you cut ties with your overweight friends! Instead of going out to eat, plan social activities. You'll have more fun together and burn calories instead of packing them on.

She also suggested that eating quickly, taking big bites or eating while watching TV, all add up to overeating.

Tip! When you attend a late night party, eat something healthy at your regular dinner time at home, like a salad or soup, before you leave home.

Caution At late night parties, in order to please the host, one has to eat but do so in small portions. Think that tomorrow is an important day at office and you have to look good which could help in avoiding binging. Late night meal causes some weight increase and one has to sweat it out more the next day.

I usually put on 1 to 1.5 kg after a late night party and it took me 36 to 48 hours to come back to normal.

Equipped with above tips and tricks, let me share how to overcome cravings for some foods which are stubborn and prevent us to gain fitness.

Most tasty foods are either savoury or sweet. Both salt and sugar are very important for our health, but the problem arises when they are consumed in quantities more than required. All agricultural products have natural salt or sugar. We are so used to adding salt or sugar to our meals that we have forgotten their natural taste. It certainly does not mean that we should eat bland food. However, we need to be aware of products that have excess of sugar or salt and they should be consumed sparingly.

Chaats: This is my favourite food. I used to have it sometimes even for lunch or dinner. The most difficult task was to control the craving for this snack. I used to eat fast and hence overate. The first thing that I did was I began to eat slowly, keeping the food longer in my mouth. This made me feel satisfied even with the lesser quantity I consumed. Mostly, chaats are considered as junk food, but they have some healthy ingredients too. I began with eating more of the healthy ones. For example, I would ask for more potatoes and curd (dahi) and less paapdi in my dahi-paapdi chat. I will take half of a samosa and more chana or *matar* in the samosa chat. This way I could eat healthy and control the cravings for my favourite foods at the same time. When I felt full, I ordered for a few pani puris. Order only one plate and share it with your friend or spouse.

Pickles: I used to eat pickles in sizable portions. My mother, and later my wife, made a variety of pickles and I hardly ate any meal without them. The salt content in pickles is so high that it leads to a lot of water absorption. Firstly, it took a huge effort to stop having a pickle as a part of my dinner, and then to replace it with something freshly made like chopped onions with green chili, garlic and lime with a little salt or any other freshly made chutney with seasonal produce. Slowly, when that experiment was successful, I applied it to my lunch meal too. Later, I restricted the use of chutneys, etc., to weekends only.

Soda drinks: I was never fond of them but I know of the addiction to soda drinks from one of my friends. She prefered a soda to any other drink and there is no limit to the quantity. On seeing how fit I was, she decided to get rid of soda first, but could not do it. It requires a strong will power. You must stop keeping a soda bottle in the refrigerator. Whenever you crave for a refreshing drink, choose a fresh lime juice or any other fresh fruit juice over soda as a healthy alternative.

> **Tip!** You must always think how to substitute the current food habit with a healthy one or something less harmful to start with.

Sweets: My other soft corner is for sweets, preferably Bengali sweets. Sweets inside the refrigerator are the biggest culprit as they are always in sight as soon as you open the door. It is always better to buy a small quantity that can be consumed immediately. But I could not enforce this rule on the rest of my family because only I was the conscious one about fitness. So, to ban or not have sweets in the refrigerator was ruled out. To resist the temptation of sweets had been a herculean task. To avoid the sight of the box of sweets in the refrigerator, I tried not to open it myself but asked other members of the family to take things out for me. After a few months, they were fed up of this system and agreed to reduce the quantity and frequency of sweets kept inside the refrigerator. I tried a few things during the initial days, like squeezing the syrup of the rasgulla to the maximum and then eating it. For other Bengali sweets where the tasty creamy part is sandwiched like breads, I removed the cream and ate the rest. It gave some satisfaction to the craving for sugar. Slowly, when I got used to it, I began to eat sweets occasionally.

Ice creams: Much before the fitness bug bit me, I had controlled eating ice cream. It was not my will power but I was afraid that I might get a sore throat. I was suggested to drink lukewarm water after eating an ice cream to avoid a sore throat. My main challenge was to control myself during parties where ice creams were always one of the desserts. Some of the flavours of ice creams are irresistible. The only way to control the intake of ice creams was to reduce the number of scoops and fill the plate of dessert with fruits. Some folks have a habit of going out with friends or families for ice creams after dinner. As said earlier, there must be a minimum of 2.5 hours gap between your last meal and sleep, so even if you indulge yourself in a bowl of ice cream occasionally, follow this rule or eat it before late afternoon. This rule could be broken occasionally to have it post dinner, but then, if you treat an ice cream a second dinner, it is no longer healthy.

Alcohol: I am not a regular drinker. So, I did not face challenges to refrain from drinking. According to many studies, moderate alcohol intake is certainly beneficial for health as even many medicines have alcohol in them. However, frequent not moderate consumption poses a challenge to fitness unless it is well-compensated with a good diet and exercise. The challenge is not just alcohol, as it does not come alone. At times, it is mixed with soda. Cocktails are the same thing. Eating unhealthy snacks with drinks add further to the woe. If you really want a flat tummy, you should limit the consumption of alcohol to one drink, take it with healthy food, followed with a lot of water to dilute it and make you feel full. Party-goers can drink slowly or dilute the drink with more water.

Snacks like mixtures, bhujjia, etc.: This one is mostly preferred by many to be taken with evening tea. In addition, these snacks are carried during travels also. To snack in general is not right, because you do not know how much you are eating. You also eat it at odd hours. I used to snack mostly in the evening or late afternoon. The first step I took was to replace it with homemade stuff like puffed rice mixed with some peanuts and a little mustard oil. This helped me to replace the unhealthy snack with a healthy one and then to remove it completely from my daily diet, leave it to be indulged occasionally.

> **Tip!** There is always a healthy or unhealthy component in tasty foods or drinks. Eat the unhealthy portion in the initial days. Slowly reduce it to a bare minimum, which can be difficult to achieve on day one. Set an intermediate diet change plan. This is better than going for an extreme schedule from day one.

It has taken me around two years to fine tune my diet. I did it slowly but steadily, and I am happy to have achieved it. Certainly, it could be done faster too, but as I wanted to make a permanent change, which is sustainable, it took me more time. I am a morning person, and here is my typical diet plan. This schedule depends upon your office timings or other outings including lunches, dinners, parties, discussions over coffee or tea, etc. If you stop doing anything suddenly, say adding sugar to your tea, the inevitable question will be, 'Are you a diabetic?' or if you stopped having deep-fried foods, you will be asked, 'Oh! Is your cholesterol high?' Isn't this how people would react? Don't mind them. You can choose to reduce the intake or stop it. As I take everything in moderate proportions, the question I am asked is how am I able to control myself.

Here is my normal meal schedule in a typical day:

Getting up time:

Drink a glass of water soaked overnight with some fenugreek (methi), cumin (jeera), coriander (*dhania*) and fennel seeds before going to restroom. Fenugreek helps in digestion. Antioxidant present in cumin seeds help in getting rid of toxic materials in the body. Coriander helps in digestion and enhances immunity. Fennel seeds increase metabolism and is a natural appetite suppressant. All of these help in weight loss.

Breakfast between 6:30 a.m.–7:00 a.m.

Oatmeal with flaxseeds and jaggery
Glass of milk
Ginger tea
Fruit
Sprouts
Soaked Almond and dry grapes

Morning drink at 9 a.m.:

Coffee with 1 healthy biscuit

Morning snack at 11 a.m.:

1 fruit

Lunch at 12:30 p.m.

Dal with 1 teaspoon of ghee
2 phulkas
Curd/raita
Cooked vegetable
Rice
Chicken (occasional)

Early afternoon beverage at 2 p.m.:

Coffee with 1 healthy biscuit

Late afternoon snack at 3:30 p.m.:

Some Fruit (occasional)

After gym meal at 6:30 p.m.:

1 full egg and 3 egg whites
2 prunes
2 dates
Sattu drink
Glass of milk

Dinner at 7:45 p.m.:

Bowl of salad
2 phulkas
Dal with one teaspoon of ghee
Cooked vegetable

> **Caution** There is a prevalent habit and a feeling that after having followed a strict weekday schedule let us treat ourselves with some 'good' food over the weekend. We self-praise, self-evaluate our efforts and treat ourselves

with unhealthy food. It is a general observation that most of the tasty food is unhealthy. In the initial stage of the fitness regime, one should try to eat it latest by evening. After progressing in the regime, you know your body and its rate of metabolism. So, you can try to eat anything in moderation, as by then the word moderation is well understood. There is nothing forbidden, but just keep in mind that everything comes at a cost. It will be painful to see that you have lost the greater part of the benefit you gained during the week and ate wrong over the weekend. As will power is not strong for many, it is better that a close friend or spouse should keep a watch on this. I know this will rob the fun, but it does work.

Protein, carbohydrate and fat are all important. It is interesting to note how our parents ate everything and they are still mostly fine, but the same is not true for later generations. What you eat needs to be balanced by physical activities.

> **Caution** Do not miss breakfast, lunch or dinner. Do not say no to fat or carbohydrate, check with doctor or dietitian if in doubt.

Then there are things like high-protein diet or low carbohydrate diet, etc. I have never tried it, so cannot comment on it. Please clear all the doubts regarding benefits and side effects before you follow such recommendations.

It is normally advisable for gym goers to focus on protein for building muscles. Protein intake should be as many grams as the weight in kgs. So, if I weigh 70 kg, I need to take a minimum 70 g of protein. For bodybuilding, the maximum amount of protein should be at most 2 times the weight in grams. I was advised to take at least 100 g and it became a challenge for me. I have tried a few things over time like increasing the number of egg whites from one to four and adding chicken in my lunch menu. But, I was never very particular about the quantity of protein and consumed what I felt was right.

> **Tip!** Make sure that breakfast, lunch and dinner all have protein in some form.

Carbohydrate is the major part of any meal and it is there for a purpose. It is the major source of energy for all activities. Carbohydrates are found in many foods. Healthy carbohydrates are found in minimally processed grains, fruits, beans, vegetables, etc., and they should always be preferred over less healthy carbs.

Fat is also good for the body as it plays a key role in keeping the body healthy. The age-old ghee—one spoon in the morning and one spoon in the evening—is always in my diet and is very helpful. It is difficult to distinguish between good fat (unsaturated ones) and bad fat. As a thumb rule, natural fat is always better.

I always believe if you are physically active and eat in moderation, you do not have to worry about the type of food you consume. It is important to have a balanced diet and slowly reduce the quantity of food. You do not need so much food, which the food industry is trying to push on us. Most of the food is deposited as fat because our body does not need it. Animals store fat to provide them energy when food is scarce and that is true for the human body too. As there is no scarcity of food for us, the fat that is deposited does not burn out. We do not hibernate as some animals do. So, what is the use of this stored fat? Nothing! It serves no purpose other than being a source of many diseases. So, why spend so much money eating things your body does not need? Why not divert that money towards physical activities? You tell me which of the two options sounds better.

SPECIAL SECTION #1

Fitness and Diet

RASHMI CHERIAN
Founder of Wellness Vows, Registered Dietician, Certified Sports and Exercise Nutritionist and a National Health Award-Winning Sports Nutritionist

Healthy eating or healthy diet is the foundation for a healthy and well-functioning body. Making changes in diet is one of the easiest ways to be fit and healthy. Healthy eating doesn't mean that you have to follow some strict diet, but to eat the right amount of healthy foods. You can be in the best shape and physically active to your maximum potential.

Majority of you struggle with healthy eating or trying to restrict random foods in your diet because:

1. Your colleagues make fun of you for being a big girl/guy in office.
2. May be your doctor wants you to shed weight to correct certain medical conditions.
3. You gained weight post-delivery and you want to get back in shape.
4. You have a family history of medical conditions (diabetes, heart problems, etc.), so you want to stay away from them.

Whatever are your reasons, please remember you are not alone. All of us struggle every day, as majority of people don't know what healthy eating means or what it means to eat a well-balanced diet to stay fit. Especially, in today's world, we are bombarded with new research every day or conflicting food advices from friends, relatives, novice trainers and coaches, who further confuse us about what we should eat. We are also often told to cut off some foods, which might help temporarily but is difficult to continue with for a longer term.

In our hectic schedule, we generally end up eating as per our convenience instead of what is healthy.

So healthy eating doesn't have to be complicated, overly restrictive, unrealistically thin, going on a zero carb or no fat diet, but it is about feeling good, having more energy and stamina with stabilized mood. It is more basic than you think. So, let us see what healthy eating or a healthy diet means.

What is Healthy Diet?

Healthy diet means a balanced diet, including:

1. Complex carbohydrates, high-quality proteins, good fats, vitamins, minerals and water.
2. Replacing processed foods with real natural ones and minimizing trans and saturated fats, alcohol and smoking.
3. Consuming right calories considering how active you are.

Healthy Eating Pyramid

The Department of Nutrition, Harvard School of Public Health launched the latest healthy eating pyramid. The widest bottom part includes the foods which are very important, whereas, foods in the narrow part need to be consumed sparingly.

The Healthy Eating Pyramid

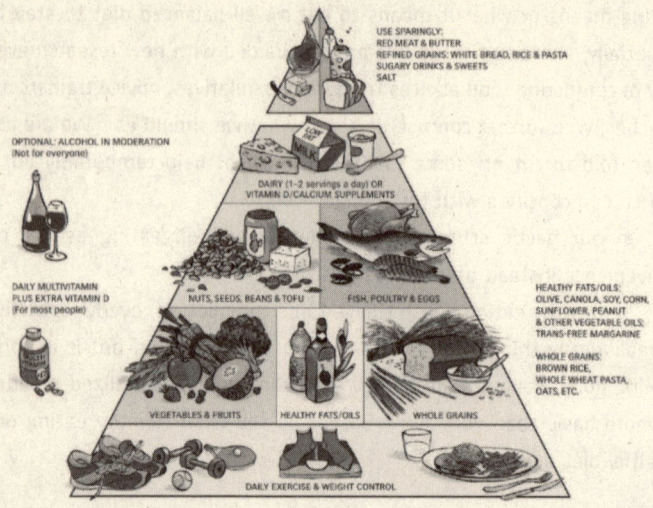

Source: Department of Nutrition, Harvard School of Public Health

How to Build a Healthy Diet

All of us need a balanced diet except for few exceptional diets that require certain restrictions. We need to learn to select healthy options from each group of foods.

Carbohydrates

Carbohydrates are the main source of energy required for physical activity, brain functioning and other bodily operations. According to the Mayo Clinic, about 45 to 65 per cent of your total daily calories should come from carbohydrates, especially if you exercise. According to the United States Department of Agriculture (USDA), the best carbohydrates are those that contain a lot of fibre, like vegetables, fruits and whole grains. They are called Complex Carbohydrates, whereas those coming from white breads, cakes, doughnuts, etc., are termed as Refined Carbs, which are also known as 'bad' carbs. Try to focus on complex unrefined carbs and stay away from simple carbs.

Guidelines for Daily Carbohydrate Intake

	SITUATION	CARBOHYDRATES TARGETS
Light	Low Intensity activities	3-5 g/kg BW per day
Moderate	Moderate Exercise (1 hr/day)	5-7 g/kg BW per day
High	Endurance (moderate to high intensity exercise of 1-3 hr/day)	7-12 g/kg BW per day
Very high	Extreme Exercise (moderate to high intensity exercise of >4-5 hr/day)	10-12 g/kg BW per day

Source: Adapted from 'The Complete Guide to Sports Nutrition' 7th ed. A. Bean.

Carbohydrate loading

Also known as Carbo or Carb Loading, it is a dietary practice used by endurance athletes like runners to increase glycogen reserves in muscle tissues and liver through the consumption of extra quantities of high-starch foods in order to improve athletic performance.

Carb Loading increases the delay in muscle fatigue by about 20 per cent and improves performance by about 2-3 per cent.

Carb Loading is considered ONLY if:

1. High-intensity endurance activity is involved where heavy demands are placed on glycogen stores.
2. Activity involves >90 minutes of continuous exercise like marathon, triathlon, etc.
3. Carbohydrate consumption is less than 7-8 g/kg of body weight per day.

Carb Loading is NOT required if:

1. The exercise is not an endurance activity.
2. Activity is <60-80 minutes like 5 km or 10 km running, short distance swimming, etc.
3. The activity is high-intensity for a short duration and will be negatively affected by the weight gain associated with loading.
4. Carbohydrate consumption is >8-9 g/kg of body weight per day.

How to carb load?

According to the Australian Institute of Sport, you should deplete for 3 to 4 days by eating a low-carb diet, then load for three to four days. During this load, you need around 7-12 g of carbohydrate per kilogram of body weight each day.

The traditional method is tapered training accompanied by high carbohydrate consumption

Foods for carb loading

1. **Grains:** Rice (brown/white/red), quinoa, oatmeal, pasta and bread.
2. **Fruits:** Berries, bananas, kiwis, sapotas, oranges, etc.
3. **Vegetables:** Potatoes, corns, squashes, yams and carrots.
4. **Nuts and Dry Fruits:** Almonds, peanuts, cashews, dates, figs, raisins, etc.
5. **Legumes:** Black beans, kidney beans, lentils, etc.

Make sure to carb load and not fat load.

Proteins

Proteins are required for body growth in kids, muscle building and repair. They are used as a source of energy when carbohydrates are depleted. You should aim for 0.8 g/kg body weight as per Recommended Dietary Allowance (RDA) if you are not very active.

For people who are into physical activities of 30-40 minutes, four to five times a week with strength training, should try to eat 1.2 to 2 g/kg body weight per day.

Protein sources

Proteins are made up of 20 amino acids, out of which nine are essential amino acids, which the body cannot make. Proteins are found in different foods, but the amount present in one kind of food varies from another. So apart from quantity, the *quality* of protein is very important and that depends upon the amino acids present in any kind of food. Therefore, proteins are divided into two groups depending upon the combinations of amino acids:

- **High Biological Value Proteins:** These proteins have essential amino acids in the same proportion required by the body, and these are obtained from animal sources like eggs, chicken, fish, meat, milk, cheese and yogurt.
- **Low Biological Value Proteins:** In these proteins, one or more of the essential amino acids are missing or present in low amount. Plant protein sources like beans, lentils, sprouts, chickpeas, legumes, nuts, seeds, etc., have low biological value proteins.

The Biological Value of Some Proteins

FOOD	BIOLOGICAL VALUE
Whey Protein Concentrate	104
Whole Egg	100
Whole Soy Bean	96
Cow Milk	91
Cheese	84
Quinoa	83
Fish	76
Whole Wheat	64
White Flour	41

In India, our diets are predominantly full of carbs. Rice is a staple component in meals in the Indian cuisine. Additionally, flat breads (chapatti, *phulka*, roti, naan, puri, etc.) made with a variety of wheat flour also make our meals high in carbs. Generally, our diets are low in proteins as the amount of dal, curd, lentils or non-veg items are very low, or they are accompanied with high carb veggies like potatoes, carrots, etc. Some of the dishes are thickened with corn or other flours, which again increases the content of carbs.

So, in order to increase proteins in our diet, few things can be done:

1. Include more of low fat cheese, curd, milk and paneer in simple forms instead of going for milk desserts (which contain added sugar and other ingredients), thick gravies, etc.
2. Include some or the other protein sources, along with rice or flatbreads, like beans, lentils, thick dals, chicken, fish or eggs in each meal.
3. Oats can be a good breakfast or snack option instead of always going for idli or dosa or different rice varieties. Oatmeal can be made interesting and delicious by adding chia seeds, flaxseeds, some chopped nuts and dry fruits.
4. Instead of high carb snacks like samosa and pakora try to opt for boiled chana chaat or bhel with sprouts or soyabean/chana cutlets, etc.
5. The same common foods can be modified a little to make them high protein. For example, a regular dosa can be made with mix of dals and lentils or sprouts (like moong dal dosa or sprouts dosa, etc.); rice can be mixed with sprouts or paneer or soy nuggets along with veggies to make one complete meal.
6. When it comes to non-veg items, consume chicken, eggs, fish, etc., in a healthy way instead of opting for kababs, fried starters, thick gravies, etc., as it just adds calories to your meal. Try to opt for tandoor, tikka, grilled and sautéed options.

Protein supplements

Protein shakes or supplements are good if they are taken along with a balanced meal to make up for the total protein intake. They are dietary supplements and completely nutritional; unlike steroids they *do not* affect our hormones. If protein powders are consumed within the actual requirement of an individual and are not abused, these supplements can turn out to be really good to meet extra protein demands, especially for an athlete to fuel any exercise or sport.

These protein powders are made from different foods like:

- Milk—Whey and casein
- Soy
- Egg
- Pea
- Hemp
- Rice

Healthy Fats

Fats are not enemies if you choose them wisely. Fats are important to produce energy, to keep you warm and to form cells and hormones. Fats also help to absorb Vitamin A, D, E and K.

About 20–25 per cent of total calories should come from healthy fats. So, what are healthy fats or good fats?

Good fats are important to produce good cholesterol and to keep heart diseases at bay, whereas bad fats produce bad cholesterol and increase the risk of cardiac problems.

Let's take a look at the different types of good and bad fats.

Good fats

- **Monounsaturated Fats:** They are found in avocados, lean meats, olive oil and nuts.
- **Polyunsaturated Fats:** Common sources of Polyunsaturated Fatty Acid

(PUFA) are plant and animal foods, such as salmon, vegetable oils and some nuts and seeds. PUFA includes Omega 3 and Omega 6 fatty acids.

- **Omega 3 sources:** Fish (tuna, salmon and mackerel), walnuts, soy foods, legumes, etc.
- **Omega 6 sources:** Vegetable oils like sunflower, peanut, canola and soy oils.

Bad fats

- **Saturated Fats:** They are found in meat fats, cream, butter, palm oil, coconut oil, etc.
- **Trans Fats:** You will find them in margarine, shortenings, doughnuts, French fries, cakes, chips, etc.

Fat as exercise fuel

Moderate to intense training requires both carbohydrates and fats. Fat supplies >50 per cent of energy during light and moderate exercises. In prolonged exercise, stored fats provide >80 per cent of energy. Overall, use of fat during exercise depends on the intensity, duration and training experience.

Fat is an extremely important nutrient in an athlete's diet because of the following reasons:

1. It keeps you full as each gram of fat provides 9 kcal unlike carbs and proteins which provide only 4 g. For people with a good appetite, struggling for high calorie demands good fat dense foods.
2. Omega 3 fatty acids prevent inflammation, which in turn reduces chances of injury.
3. PUFA maintain a balance in steroid hormones, which is important for athletic performance and recovery.

Fibre

Fibre helps to prevent heart diseases, diabetes, weight gain, cancers, etc. Depending on age and gender, nutrition experts recommend at least 21 to 38 grams of fibre each day for optimal health. We get fiber from oats, whole-wheat flour, wheat bran, fruits, vegetables, beans, etc.

For athletes, prior to any competition or event, avoid a high-fibre meal as it may cause an upset stomach. Prefer a low-fibre food like white rice, potatoes without skin, etc.

Water and hydration

Water is very important for good health and the requirements vary from individual to individual depending upon environment, health, how active they are, etc. According to the Food and Nutrition Board of the Institute of Medicine, water intake recommendation for men is 3.7 litres daily, while women should aim for 2.7 litres. Always remember this measurement need not come only from drinking water, but will include water from food and other beverages.

Exercise or any physical activity increases fluid demands in the body. When the body works hard, more heat is produced which in turn needs to be lost. As a result more fluids are required. As a rule, 500–750 ml per hour of water needs to be consumed in addition to the above-mentioned requirements. This varies from person to person.

The best way to estimate how much fluid you lose during exercise is to weigh yourself before and after an hour of exercise. For every 1 kg of weight you lose, you have lost approximately 1 litre of fluid from your body.

More fuilds are required for more than 90 minutes of moderate to high-intensity exercises and in such cases a sports drink is a must with 6 per cent glucose solution to replenish glycogen stores and to maintain steady energy levels.

When to drink water?

- On Waking up
  - Drink water as soon as you wake up as your body is slightly dehydrated

- Pre-exercise
  - Drink 5–7 ml per kg of body weight at least 4 hours before the session. So for a 55 kg athlete, this would be 275 ml–385 ml
  - Weigh yourself immediately before you begin your workout.
- During Exercise
  - Aim to replace 80 per cent of losses whilst exercising.
  - During long events, it is suggested to keep sipping fluids. Drink one cup of water every 15 minutes. Frequent small sips also prevent bloating.
- Post-exercise
  - It is very important to drink fluids immediately post an event to replenish body fluids and to flush out metabolic wastes.
  - Consume as much fluids as tolerated. An intake of 250 ml per 15 minutes needs to be maintained for the next 3 hours.
  - Fluids should contain both carbohydrates and electrolytes.

Dehydration

It occurs when the body loses more fluids than it takes in. As a result, the amount of blood in your body decreases which strains the heart, lungs and circulatory system. Dehydration as low as 2 per cent can impair performance.

Effects of Dehydration

PER CENT WEIGHT LOSS (kg)	EFFECTS ON THE BODY
1–2	Increase in core body temperature
3	Significant increase in body temperature with aerobic exercise
5	<ul><li>Significant increase in body temperature with definite decrease in aerobic ability and muscular endurance</li><li>Possible 20–30 per cent decrease in strength and anaerobic power</li><li>Susceptibility to heat exhaustion</li></ul>

6	Muscle spasms, cramping
10 or more	- Excessively high core body temperature
- Susceptibility to heat stroke
- Heat injury and circulatory collapse with aerobic performance

Source: Alabama A&M and Auburn Universities, 2003.

Note: With a 5 per cent body weight loss, an athlete will need at least 5 hours to rehydrate.

Where Do the Calories Fit In?

All the foods we eat contain calories. The more calories you eat, the more energy is supplied to the body. Total calorie intake for an individual depends on a lot of factors like age, gender, height, weight, lifestyle, medical conditions (if any) and general health.

As per the RDA for Indians, a reference adult sedentary man (60 kg) can consume 2,300 calories, whereas women (55 kg) can consume 1,900 calories.

For more accurate calorie calculations as per the physical activity, Basal Metabolic Rate (BMR) is multiplied with a number (which represents physical activity) and that final number is the total calorie requirement for an individual.

Sedentary – BMR x 1.2

Moderate – BMR x 1.55

Active – BMR x .725

Very Active – BMR x 1.9

Foods to Fuel Workouts

Workout or sports nutrition is very important to get results on the court or in a gym and for performance and recovery.

PRE-workout nutrition

A good pre-workout meal can make a huge difference in overall performance and recovery.

1-3 hours before workout

Ideally, a meal should be consumed 1-3 hours prior to the workout or competition depending upon how well you can tolerate food. Some of the pre-workout meal suggestions are:

- Bread with peanut butter
- Yogurt with berries
- Breakfast cereals with milk
- Whole wheat pasta with veggies

60 minutes to 1 hour before workout

- Veggies with hummus
- Fruits: Banana, berries, etc.
  - Nuts and Dry Fruits
  - Energy Bars

DURING workout nutrition

During a workout, nutrition is important for hydration, to keep energy levels up, preserve muscles and boost performance.

Some options include:

- Coconut Water
- Water
- Sports Drink or gel
- Banana
- Salted Nuts
- Energy Bars

POST-workout nutrition

Post-workout meal is important for rehydration, recovery, muscle building and repair. The hour, immediately after a workout, called the 'golden hour', is the time when the muscles are craving for proteins and nutrients. This meal is very important for replenishing energy sources.

Some of the foods, which can be included in a post-workout meal, are below:

- Protein shake
- Low fat chocolate milk
- Egg whites
- Buttermilk
- Yogurt
- Chicken or fish with veggies and mashed potatoes
- Fruit shake or smoothie
- Rasgulla (squeezed and washed in water)
- Cereals with skimmed milk

Why is Eating Healthy Important for Overall Fitness?

So far we have learnt what to eat and how to eat healthy to keep fit. To conclude, let's now take a look at why this is necessary.

- Good nutrition improves immunity. When we eat a healthy balanced meal, our body is able to fight sicknesses and illnesses in a better way making us stronger.
- Smart food choices protect from chronic diseases like hypertension, cardiac problems, etc.
- Children who have healthy eating habits have good cognitive function. and they perform well in academics and sports both.
- Healthy eating improves stamina and endurance.
- It saves money.

- It reduces stress.
- It improves fertility.
- It reduces cravings.

Top Super Foods for Fitness

Below are some super foods, which when incorporated regularly, will not only help in good fitness but in good health.

1. Avocado: Avocadoes are rich in mono and polyunsaturated fats, which help to lower bad cholesterol and promote lean muscle growth. It is also an anti-inflammatory food.
2. Chicken: Chicken is a source of high-quality protein and essential amino acids which when consumed post-workout along with veggies will help in muscle building and repair.
3. Eggs: Eggs contain a plethora of vitamins and minerals along with high biological value proteins. It contains healthy fats for the heart and brain. It supports muscle growth and helps in fat loss.
4. Salmon: Salmon is rich in omega 3, which helps in building muscles, post-workout recovery and reduces soreness in muscles.
5. Beets: Beets contains nitrates, which increases inflow of oxygen to the muscles. A glass of beetroot juice 1–1.5 hours before a session or run will enhance strength, stamina and endurance.
6. Sweet Potatoes: They contain complex carbohydrates, which have low glycemic index. It digests slowly and provides energy to the body for long. It also has anti-inflammatory effect.
7. Pineapple: Pineapple heals injuries faster as it contains an enzyme named bromelain, which has anti-inflammatory effect.
8. Chocolate Milk: It is the best post-workout drink as it contains ideal carb to protein ratio essential for recovery and rehydration. It also contains magnesium, which helps in recovery.
9. Hemp seeds: They are natural appetite suppressants, which keep you full longer and avoid sugar cravings. It is full of proteins, fats,

antioxidants and other essential nutrients.
10. Turmeric: Curcumin in turmeric has anti-inflammatory effect, which protects an athlete from any damage and gives a good night sleep.
11. Ginger: Ginger helps with delayed onset muscle soreness (DOMS) as it is a pain reliever and anti-inflammatory.
12. Watermelon: Watermelon contains an amino acid L-citrulline, which helps in recovery as it helps in faster removal of lactic acid than normal.

Now that you are aware of healthy eating and nutrition intake required for fitness, it is time to start! Good nutrition is all about balance.

FIVE

Fitness through Gym

When I first entered the gym, the type and range of equipment bemused me. I wondered why so many equipment were required. With the passage of time, I learnt more about them. A lot of them are used in multiple ways to provide diverse benefits.

Gym equipment can be categorized into cardiovascular equipment and weight equipment. Treadmills, cross trainers, rowers, cycles, etc., are some examples of cardiovascular equipment.

There are dumbbells, flat benches, incline benches, steppers, mats, medicine balls, gym balls and other items coupled with an open floor space, basically, for floor exercises and endurance training.

Before we proceed to exercises, let us focus on some basic facts, which need to be kept in mind while doing any exercise:

Purpose of Hitting the Gym

You should be very clear about your purpose of joining a gym. If you are unsure about it, here are some interesting anecdotes I have gathered observing people with mixed up priorities visiting the gym:

1. **To get into shape for your wedding:** I have noticed people in my office gym as well as the one I attend. There is always a new face or a neo convert into fitness, who wants a quick result to look good. Most of the time, it is for a wedding or some important event. Sure, if the event is say half a year away, you will start to see the benefits, but when it is just a few weeks away, it is more of a ritual to check the fitness box as a pre-wedding preparation. Certainly, any gym would entertain new joiners, but no gym can actually give you results in a short time. Results will be visible if you continue for a long period. This haphazard and quick approach to fitness leads to injuries.

However, a couple of years ago, I saw one man with a fit body coming to gym a few days a week. He got along with all the trainers and it appeared that they knew him quite well. One day, I saw him helping a somewhat obese woman in her workout. He fully focused on her regime to make sure that she does it the right way. Henceforth, he came to the gym regularly to train that woman.

One day, I could not control my curiosity and asked my trainer, 'Does the gym allow external trainers to provide personal training to a gym member?'

'No sir, we do not allow it, but then one friend can help another friend and we cannot stop them from doing so.'

I pointed at the guy and asked, 'Isn't he a trainer?'

'He is a friend of that trainer and these three know each other well,' he smiled and said in a hushed voice.

'It is important that she reduces some weight soon.'

I was puzzled by this cryptic answer and stared at him. Sensing my curiosity, he continued, 'Sir, they are childhood friends and in love. She is very intelligent and qualified. The guy is also very good. They want to get married, but the guy's family want her to lose weight. So, he and the trainer both are trying very hard to help her reduce weight.'

My respect for them grew.

> **Tip!** It is excellent if a relationship can enforce dedication towards fitness, but then the fitness regime should continue for long.

I did not see them for a few months and then one day I saw them on the treadmills arguing loudly. She had reduced some weight, but I could not relate them with my older image of theirs where they hardly talked and only focused on fitness.

I was doing my warm up exercises when my trainer came to me. Their arguments also distracted him. We looked at each other and he whispered, 'Sir, they started fighting soon after their marriage.' We smiled.

'At least they are coming to the gym after marriage,' I added.

2. **To hang out with friends:** There are group of friends who come to check out a gym. They join the gym and synchronize their timing with each other's. A few are serious about fitness while the others chat, check their phones or spend more time changing the song on the gym's music system. Such uncommitted friends end up distracting the ones who are serious about their regime.

> **Caution** Gym is a temple of fitness rather than a place to hang out with friends. Those friends who are not serious

about their regime should be reminded politely to not distract the serious ones.

There is a silver lining in this too. Probably, those who join just for the heck of it might get motivated and take up fitness seriously after watching others.

Then there is another bunch of friends, where one of them is into an advance stage of fitness and he could act as a buddy for the others and motivate them. I have seen a higher level of seriousness in such a bunch of friends, because the buddy usually ensures that all of them start with their right set of exercises, because that was the reason why they are in the gym.

3. **Making new friends to hang out outside the gym:** A few are on the lookout to make some new friends. They tend to be extra friendly to strangers and spend more time to talk and help rather than do their own exercises. Over time, such a person will synchronize his or her timing with the other's to take the friendship forward. The priority should be to join the gym for fitness and not be the other way around. On the other hand, it would be nice to meet someone special. If the priority is to find a date, it should be clear in the mind, only then let fitness take a back seat. As these things do not happen immediately, make sure that you do not negate fitness as you go through such a phase.

The challenge does not stop here. You should know that not every relationship is steady and it may end sooner than expected with one dropping out of the gym. I don't know whether that person would join another gym, but it certainly affects the journey towards fitness. If the person comes with a bunch of friends, and they witness the whole thing, it becomes even more embarrassing.

> **Tip!** Inside a gym, your priority should be fitness and any other thing needs to be handled in a way that it should not affect your journey towards fitness.

4. Give gym a try: I have seen a few who are not patient to see the result of an activity that they undertake for fitness. They are always in a hurry for a quick result. They would hop from one activity to another and will be quick to decide that nothing would work for them. They come with a mindset to find the kind of activity that suits them. Whether you are into marathons, yoga, Zumba, aerobics or sports, the result will be visible in due course of time.

> **Caution** Joining a gym to try if it works for you is a wrong mindset. The right way is how you can make it work for yourself.

Excuses like genetics, insufficient time, earlier injuries, 'cannot control food', 'I look fine', etc., influence a person's thought and hinder to take up anything seriously. For all these excuses, there are ways to overcome it. Only after that can a person reap benefits from a routine.

5. Desire for quick and visible biceps: I have seen some people who come to the gym and head straight to where the weights are kept. They pick up a suitable dumbbell, go in front of a mirror and start arm curls. After a few repetitions, they will look into the mirror to check the impact on their biceps from different angles, check their phones and finally lift another dumbbell for a few more repetitions. Don't you relate to this in your own gym, or maybe you are one of them?

> **Tip!** Gym is not for standing in front of the mirror and looking at yourself for any sign of quick gain, but pledging in front of the mirror that you will change and change for good.

Whatever the purpose of joining the gym, make sure you keep fitness as the primary goal. People seeking fitness could fall into the following categories.

1. **To fix their health and weight issues:** Professionals today who spend most of their time sitting in front of a computer are deprived of sufficient exercise, and end up putting on unwanted weight (mostly fat). This affects their blood sugar and lipid profile numbers. When warning signs are visible, they take up exercise after a doctor's advice. Generally, this bunch sticks to cardio, and can be found walking/running either on the treadmill or in the local park.
2. **To seek mind-body connect, focus, spirituality, etc.:** In today's hectic lifestyle that involves a lot of work-related stress, people often are worn out even before they reach the office battling traffic. To undo this chaos and trauma, some seek refuge in our ancient techniques like yoga and meditation or join the gyms that provide such classes too.
3. **To perform daily activities better:** This sort of people want to strengthen themselves by being fit and flexible enough to handle the rigorous physical needs of daily

life or to pursue a specific hobby. The exercises could include aerobics, functional training, free body exercises and some strength training.
4. **To sculpt into Greek gods:** Yes, there is nothing wrong to aspire for a sculpted and awesome physique. Having a well-sculpted body is an asset that can boost your confidence tremendously. It also comes with a 'good' side effect of health! Not surprisingly, this category of people is seen mostly at the weights section of the gym pumping away as they admire the awesomeness of their bodies in front of the mirror.

> **Tip!** Plan a fitness regime by jotting down the objectives and the target date. Failing to plan will mean planning to fail! Keep the expectations within limits of sanity. It must have taken you years to go out of shape, so you need to be patient to get back in shape, and there is no shortcut to it.

Now let's look at some other aspects that you must keep in mind while doing the exercises.

Gym Etiquettes

Gym has some etiquettes which when followed will help you and might help other gym members too.

1. **Proper attire and hygiene:** The first thing that you should choose before going to a gym is the right shoes. Shoes should be comfortable and good for brisk walking or running so that your feet are fine while doing any cardiovascular exercises. Bring your shoes rather than wearing them to the gym, as they will soil the gym. Your choice of gym outfit should be somewhat loose

to help in easy body movement, air circulation and to facilitate sweating. Cotton should be preferred, but then there are some quality synthetic materials, which are made for workouts exclusively. Choose accordingly and as per the season. Some people do not use deodorants and it gets worse when they exercise wearing sleeveless t-shirts, which is disgusting for other members. Use a mild deodorant, as a strong one hinders too. Keeping a towel handy is another thing that will help you in taking care of the sweat and stopping it from falling onto the benches and other areas used during your session.

> **Caution** Wipe the area of the gym equipment, which has come into your contact to help other gym members use it hygienically.

2. **Use of weights and other paraphernalia:** How do you feel if you search a particular set of dumbbells and you do not find it at its place? You search the whole gym and find one of them at one place and the other one at another. Irritated? Many do not even consider keeping the dumbbell back in its place. It is true for mats, steppers, medicine balls, skipping ropes and the list goes on. It is a prevalent mindset that the person who takes care of the gym should do these things. But at peak hours, it is not at all possible for any one person to put things back to where they belong, causing inconvenience to other members.
3. **Ogling other gym members:** I have observed some of the new entrants of the gym ogle others who are fit. A cursory glance is fine, but a constant stare and sometimes standing near that person and watching is not the right

behaviour. The reason to ogle could be anything, but make sure that you do not make others uncomfortable. In my initial days, I used to observe, not stare, at a couple of them to set some goal and strengthen my mind to take up certain exercises. In the last few years, I am now on the other side of the spectrum where, occasionally, I am being stared at.

However, it is wrong to stare at someone even if you want to learn the right posture to do an exercise. You could reach out and take inputs from him or her or ask some trainer to help you. It might be better if you could also inform him or her in advance that you would want to watch some of the postures. Understand that your body is different from the other person's and you are at a different stage in the fitness journey. So your needs are different and cannot be copied from that person.

4. **Showing off:** This habit is a disruptive and impolite act, which others do not seek. It is not about flaunting your body; it is not about sharing the progress with your friends and comparing exercises and muscle growth. It is about doing it in a way so that it does not distract others. One person joined my gym for a short duration. He had a well-maintained physique. He usually did heavy weights and had a peculiar habit of looking around after each set. I don't know whether he did that to simply seek appreciation or try to initiate a conversation with someone. After each set, he would go near other members who were busy with their exercise. I could see some get irritated with his behaviour and the trainers felt helpless as they could not ask him to stop. One day, he changed his exercise, and started talking to himself loudly while lifting a heavy weight.

'Come on, baby,' would be his first sentence while lifting the weight and towards the end of the set, when it becomes more difficult he would say, 'Come on, baby, you can't deny me.'

Tip! Keep a proper decorum inside the gym. This is important as a courtesy to fellow members.

5. **Warm up and stretches:** When I joined the gym, I had heard many times that a proper warm up before starting the exercise and stretches after the exercise is very important. Honestly speaking, I had never taken it seriously. This was because it seemed like a waste of time and a tactic my trainer used. I wanted to jump into the main exercise quickly. Moreover, during the warm up, I was asked to rotate my shoulders, stretch my legs and arms, bend over to touch my feet and so on, which I thought was of little use. Initially, I did not know that the low-speed walking on the treadmill was also a part of the warm-up routine. I was also not serious about the stretches at the end of the routine.

In the beginning, I did not face any problems from the fewer warm-ups and stretches. As time passed and I became more aware of a fitness routine, I understood the importance of it, but still did not take it seriously. Over the years, I met a few fitness freaks who had injured themselves due to the lack of proper stretches after the exercises. I too got concerned about possible injuries and began to focus on stretches to avoid them.

One fine day, my new physiotherapist-cum-trainer who was quite strict told me in the presence of my regular trainer, 'So far your progress was gradual as you were doing moderate exercises. These new exercises, which I am suggesting are above the moderate level, and your body is ready to take them up. You will be doing full body weights one day and endurance exercises the next day.'

'As I will not monitor your progress on a daily basis, please make sure you do not miss on 10-minutes stretches after the workout. You must take care of your lower back and hamstrings,' he continued. This was a thinly veiled warning.

I began to feel the stress on both areas—lower back and hamstrings—after doing the new exercises. The stretches did help me. Finally, I was fully brought into this concept of warm-ups and stretches and started to take it very seriously. It is very important that you focus on these to avoid any injury.

6. **Music:** Music is a very important aspect during exercise. It not only breaks monotony, but the beat of the music also pumps up and motivates you to do better. You can carry your own collection and exercise with headphones on, while others listen to the gym's music system. Sometime members play their own collection of music in the gym. I like the variety of music and anything from soothing to hard rock, provided the genre keeps changing, which breaks the rhythm and monotony.

    Fast-paced music is usually played at the gym to get the adrenaline pumping. Listening to music can help make the otherwise boring treadmill session interesting. So, if you are someone who loves your music during the workout, carry your headphones, preferably a wireless/Bluetooth model. I do not use headphones, because they hinder the mind-body connect; the gym music system instead works better for me. You may use the latter too.

A new member joined and was assigned the same trainer as mine. She was doing warm-ups. The usual gym music was on but at a low volume. Suddenly, a devotional song started blaring near my workout area, startling everyone. People were puzzled about the source of this music, which happened to be her mobile. She continued with her exercises but then suddenly the music stopped due to an incoming call. She went out to take the call.

Her trainer looked at me and said, 'This is the first time in my decade-long career that I have come across such a person.' She came back but did not put on her music and focused on the remaining warm-up routine.

Tip! It is important to keep changing the music collection, be it personal or at the gym to avoid the monotony and predictability of the song, thereby inducing excitement and boosting motivation to exercise better.

7. **Mirrors:** The inside walls of a gym are mostly mirrors. They are especially helpful to keep a check on your posture and to correct them. It also serves as a place for fitness enthusiasts to look at themselves during and between sets—admiring the change brought about by their hard work. It is fine to be a little obsessed with yourself when it comes to fitness, as miracles can be achieved with a little obsession.

Eating Before the Gym

It is debatable if you can exercise empty stomach or not. You need to eat light before a workout. The food that you eat at night gets digested and you wake up with an empty stomach. Occasionally, I was told to have a glass of milk and one banana before I go to the gym in the morning. This is light enough to exercise even within 30 minutes of eating and is sufficient to provide energy to undertake exercises.

Initially, I did feel dizzy while doing the exercises in the morning. But by taking proper food and with the body getting used to the regime, the dizziness stopped. If you feel dizzy, stop the exercise and take some rest. Do as per your comfort in the first week and gradually increase from second. If you still feel uneasy, do not push yourself, but listen to your body.

However, it totally depends on a person's comfort level with working out on an empty stomach. Coffee (punches a good caffeine boost) or just plain water works for some. For some people, a light to moderate level of exercise is manageable with the glycogen stores in the body from the previous night's meal. However, some of them feel exhausted and are unable to give their 100 per cent, especially if the routine is intense. They need some kind of pre-workout meal. Slow digesting carbohydrates and proteins are ideal ingredients in a pre-workout meal. Some of the good pre-workout foods are egg whites, milk, oats, banana and peanut butter sandwich.

As the morning is premium and the digestion of a pre-workout meal will be somewhere between 30 minutes to 90 minutes, some take fast digesting whey protein to save time.

Caution Know your body to decide your pre-workout meal. If in doubt, it is better to take a light one. It is not true that exercising on an empty stomach burns fat. Human body is a complex machine. When and how much the body uses the energy sources, i.e., consumed food, stored fat, muscle (the body breaks down muscle for energy) is a complex subject.

It is easier in the evening to workout as you eat throughout the day, but the key is how much food you have consumed and how many hours before the workout you have had the food. About 2–3 hours after lunch is fine, but if the lunch was slightly heavy, 3–4 hours will be better. If you are going for a late evening workout, take one fruit or some hot beverage with a biscuit. Doing the exercise on a heavy stomach will not give you the desired result other than aiding digestion and burning some calories. If you really want to reduce weight, your calorie intake should be less and the exercises should help in burning the excess.

Eating After the Gym

It is important to supply the body with essential nutrients, especially after an intense and draining workout at the gym to replenish energy stores and rebuild damaged tissues. A good mix of protein and carbohydrates are needed after the workout. Avoid delaying or missing a meal. Those who take supplements like whey protein shakes need to take it after the workout also for faster absorption.

Eating after exercise is very important. This is the time your muscles need protein and that too fast. I normally eat within 30 minutes of completing my exercise.

Importance of Sleep

After nutrition, the next important requirement is adequate sleep. In fact, lack of sleep is said to cause more disastrous effects to one's physical and mental health when compared to lack of adequate nutrition and water. Hence, it makes sense for fit and not-so-fit people alike, to give their body at least 6–8 hours of sleep. Note that watching TV or WhatsApp videos while lying in bed does not count as sleep. When you sleep, the body repairs wear and tear of the muscles and rebuilds them. It is also the time that the brain flushes toxins and recharges itself; the lack of sleep can permanently damage brain cells.

There are two kinds of people when it comes to how they feel after a workout. The first group of people feels more energetic and full of life—it is best if this group works out in the morning so that they can leverage their uplifted mood throughout the day and perform their daily activities better. The second group of people seems to be hit by a speeding truck after their workout. All their energy is sapped by the intense gym session, and they are drained physically and mentally. They walk around like zombies throughout the day, and try hard not to fall asleep during meetings. It is better if this group works out in the evening, so that their daily activities are not adversely affected by a morning workout. Unless of course, they can get a good couple of hours of sleep after the post-workout meal, which is a luxury not many people have in this busy world.

Whatever group of people one falls in, everyone gets a dose of the sleepy feeling a couple of hours after the workout. However, if your schedule only permits a morning visit to the gym, don't lose hope; try to look for other ways to get some rest. A quick power-nap in the taxi on the way to office, or a few winks during lunch hour goes a long way in recharging the mind and the body.

Tip! Importance of sleep will be an under-statement. A well-rested body is the key for fitness.

Under the A/C or Fan:

If your gym has centralized A/C, there are very less options to request to increase or decrease the temperature. On the other hand, if your gym has a combination of A/Cs and fans at various locations, you have more flexibility. I have the fan or A/C switched off when I do my exercises to enable me sweat more, and when I feel uncomfortable, I exercise under the fan or have the A/C switched on.

Tip! Check your comfort level and decide whether you need an A/C or a fan, but ensure that you sweat easily.

Hydration

Why should you drink water when you sweat during a workout? The fact is you need to keep your body hydrated during exercises. When you sweat, it leads to dehydration and intake of water is very important. Some of them add glucose to it to get more energy during the exercises. It is your choice, but please keep in mind that you are also adding additional sugar to it. I take only water.

Caution Don't gulp water, but sip at it slowly while exercising.

Right Way To Exercise

Why do people lose hope of any improvement despite clocking months in gyms?

The simple answer is that they don't do the exercise in a right way. Each exercise is meant for a body part and there are some compound exercises like squats, bench presses, pull-ups, etc., which target multiple body parts. The impact of the exercise should be on the desired body part.

How will you come to know that the exercise has been done properly?

One straightforward way is through muscle soreness discussed earlier is known as DOMS, which is mostly felt 24 hours to 36 hours after the exercise. If this soreness is happening to the targeted body part, you are doing it in a right way. Muscle soreness does not happen after any regular exercise or the exercise to which your body part is accustomed. It happens when you target that part with a different or intense set of new exercise.

If you target any part of the body, say biceps or triceps, make sure to repeat the exercise not before 48 hours. As said earlier, exercise is also a mental game. Don't look into the mirror all the time or think about other things while doing the exercise in a mechanical way. Focus your mind on that part of your body that you want to target, as mind-muscle connection is very important to get the desired result.

> **Tip!** Exercise tears the muscle and the resting period of 48 hours will help the muscle to heal and grow. Focus your mind on the body part that you are targeting, to help in better blood flow.

During my initial days, I used to get tired after a few repetitions or after every set. My trainer tried a lot to reduce my rest period between sets, but he could not. Sometimes, he would pull me up from rest and join me in the exercises to cut down on my time between exercises. I was puzzled why such a hurry when I finish my exercise anyway. I hit plateau and that too for a long duration and he repeatedly advised me to reduce the waiting period between sets, but I did not pay any heed initially.

> **Tip!** A thirty-second rest between sets and 2-3 minutes rest between two exercises is an ideal one. This will ensure that your heartbeat does not come down to resting levels to provide maximum gain from the exercise.

You might have noticed that some members make a lot of noise when they pick up heavy weights. They breathe out. The more you exhale, the more you expel carbon dioxide from your body, which had accumulated in your body. Most people, who use treadmills, do not make any sound even though they too exhale carbon dioxide.

> **Tip!** For the exercise to be effective, breathe out when you exert force during any exercise and breathe in when you come back to a resting position. Even when you use a treadmill, exhale from your mouth for better results.

Another frequently asked question is about the frequency of exercises.

Since childhood my grandparents told me, which my mother always repeated, to keep the body active; the more active you are the better you will be. Laced with such *gyan*,

I was very excited to be a regular at the gym. Though that impressed my trainer, but then a few weeks later, he told me,

'Sir, it is Sunday tomorrow. Take full rest.'

'What do you mean by full rest?' I asked.

'Sir, full rest means don't try any other exercises on Sunday,' he explained.

'How can I laze around on Sunday, I will do some brisk walking,' I protested.

'No. Just do your daily chores and whatever normal walking is required, that should be sufficient. Don't do brisk walking or any other exercise. Your body needs full rest. This will help your body to prepare you well for the next week,' he explained.

Unconvincingly I took his words. Over the years, I realized how the rested body really helps and why it was told many times in the past, which I reluctantly followed.

> **Tip!** 'Listen to your body'; a well-rested body can do the exercises better than an overly tired one.

Depending upon your fitness condition, four, five or six days a week should be quite good. I still maintain a frequency of five to six days a week. If I workout fewer days in a week for any reason, there is no feeling of guilt which I experienced earlier. There are some who visit the gym 2–3 times a week only and maintain themselves well, but then they are active and follow the diet diligently.

Measuring Progress of Fitness

This is a common question asked by everyone—how to measure the progress and ascertain that you are moving in the right direction?

Most gyms provide the facility to measure progress in two ways periodically. It could be done as early as four weeks or as late as eight to twelve weeks.

Type 1: In this type of measurement, every part of the body is measured, as it provides the progress of any part shrunk or grown. Every part of the body is measured—chest exhaled and inhaled, shoulders, neck, arms normal and arms full, abs upper and abs lower, waist, hip, calves and thighs. A measuring tape is used for these measurements.

Type 2: Usually done with the earlier one, but the chest, mid-axillary, triceps, sub scapular, abdomen, super iliacus, mid-thighs, etc., are measured by calipers. These are done to calculate the total body fat percentage, lean body mass, Body Mass Index (BMI), etc.

The above two measurements are used by the trainer to decide what part of the body needs to be focused on and what type of exercise should be prescribed. Accordingly, a worksheet is made which provides the details of weekly schedule which then the trainer explains to you. Such plan is followed until the next checkup and this is how fitness is tracked.

Role of Legs in Achieving Fitness

Legs play an important part in most of the cardio exercises, and being the biggest muscles of the body like the glutes and quadriceps, they burn calories for many hours after a good and intense exercise. Any gym trainer will stress not to ignore the legs because they are less visible.

After my reduced weight started to show, I was impatient to look fit just like everyone else. I was in a dilemma on how to ask this to my trainer and every time I asked in a roundabout way, and he gave the same answer: 'I am making you do a complete body workout with more focus on cardiovascular so that your weight reduces.'

After a few such nagging questions over the weeks, he got my point and asked me pointedly, 'Oh! Which movie star do you want to look like?'

He laughed and named some of them and talked about the shape of their bodies. Towards the end he said, 'If you continue to be regular in the gym, over the years you will be more of an athletic and lean type rather than bulky and broad type. I think athletic and lean type will suit you well.'

I felt encouraged and asked, 'So, what else should I do to achieve that?'

'This is a long journey, but then the benefit of exercise comes when you exercise the most hidden part of the body—legs.'

With that, he quickly added a word of caution.

'Guys need to be careful about chicken legs. Leg exercises should be done keeping this in mind.'

Caution Avoid chicken legs, as your whole body weight falls on the legs and they should be strong enough to support it.

I verified with others and they all said the same thing. One of them even said that the actual fitness is visible only through legs. Some of the movie stars go shirtless because they probably appear fit on screen, but if one sees their legs, they might not appear so fit.

Leg exercises not only help leg muscles like quadriceps, hamstrings, calves, but they also help other muscles of the body, and normally leg exercises are recommended to be done towards the end to get better results.

> **Tip!** Legs are the most important part of the body, as leg exercises will also indirectly help the other parts of the body get stronger. Stronger legs will go a long way in maintaining the fitness.

Internet Content on Fitness

Internet is flooded with information. It is a challenge to skim through it to find what works for you and what does not. All the information available on the Internet is not always verified. If you apply online content as your fitness regime, it might pose a challenge when you are new to the gym. At the gym, you can get a holistic schedule that suits you. When in doubt, ask people and learn from their experiences. In such a process, I might have interacted with more than two dozen people inside the gym or at my office for various inputs during my journey of fitness. I have verified some of my observations. Sometimes, I have taken their inputs and discussed them with the gym trainers to ascertain what might work. At times, I have asked a few of my colleagues to check with their gym trainers on specific issues to clarify my doubt. This helped me increase my knowledge. Some people have a few favourite websites and a few favourite videos too. I also went through some of them and refined my knowledge.

Some people commented that they trust their favourite sites more than the trainers, as these sites have accumulated knowledge, whereas trainers have limited knowledge. Also, all gyms don't have certified trainers and most of them are self-trained with little experience.

> **Tip!** All sources of information are welcome, but then one has to choose wisely and apply them in the right manner.

Here I will try to make your life easy by helping you in what you should do in a given situation. In each scenario, you should keep some goal in mind and get frequently inspired by your role model. That helps you achieve the goal gradually. Depending upon your progress, a certain set of exercises should be continues for 6 weeks to 2 months, and thereafter, you should change the full exercise regime, so that the body does not get used to it. Once the body gets accustomed, the benefit of exercise will diminish the effect.

Workout Methodologies

Push-pull strategy

In this plan, the idea is to work the body parts involved in a 'push' movement one day, and work the parts that 'pull' on the another day.

- Push day includes those exercises that make the chest, shoulders and triceps workout.
- Pull day includes those exercises that make the back and biceps workout.
- The leg can be exercised on a different day. Alternatively, the push-pull theory can be applied here as well—quadriceps on push day and hamstrings on pull day.

These types are intense workouts that involve 3–4 muscles and should be coupled with light cardiovascular exercises.

If the exercise is too intense, the third day of your routine can be a light day with mild cardiovascular exercise only.

Full body, with endurance exercise in between, on alternate days

In this routine, all body parts are exercised every alternate day. Typically, one exercise type per body part, and these are changed in each session. For example, Monday for shoulder and barbell presses, Wednesday for dumbbell front raise and Friday for shrugs.

On other days, floor exercises like jumping jacks and mountain climbing are recommended, which increase endurance.

4-day, 5-day or 6-day split

This is another popular variation where typically one or two groups of muscles are exercised each day. The sessions are expected to be short, but intense and focus on a particular body part. This part of the body then gets a full week's rest from any direct work. It is also common to club smaller muscles like biceps with another body part like the back that needs to be exercised on the same day. Similarly, for someone who cannot make many trips to the gym can combine shoulder and leg days.

Higher repetitions-lower weight

Individuals who try to tone the muscles to bring more definition sometimes use this strategy. It keeps the heart rate up for a longer while working the muscles. Its effect is similar to a cardio or endurance training.

Lower repetitions-heavy weight

This strategy is used to build muscles if you are in a bulk up phase. Intense exercises, typically done until muscle failure (the point where you cannot do another repetition), causes micro-tears in the muscle fibres which repair and re-build into bigger and stronger muscles to handle the increased workload.

5 Fabulous Exercises: Recommendation Under Paucity of Time

When I am running short of time to do the exercises, or I am unable to go to the gym, I just focus on the following five exercises, which provide immense satisfaction and result. Another advantage is that these exercises mostly use the body weight as resistance and require minimum to no equipment. These exercises can be done after a break as a means to prepare the body for the rigorous strength training.

- **Pull-ups:** A very popular exercise, which many try but a few succeed to do in the right way. First, one should just try to hang properly and try to balance the body. Once you gain some confidence, try to pull your body up slowly. Initially, I used to jerk my leg to lift my body, which is a wrong thing to do and I realized this later. Thankfully, it did not cause any injury. Once you have lifted your body, try to hold it at that position and count to five before you lower your body slowly. This is the key to this exercise. Rather than focusing on number of repetitions, focus on the right posture. Some people take months to come to this level, so be patient. You can start with five and can go up to 10 or more as per your comfort level.

    This exercise is a litmus test for upper body strength.

It is the mainstay for workout routines for the back. This exercise strengthens the upper back, particularly the latissimus dorsi, popularly known as 'lats' or even 'wings'. It also improves the biceps and the strength of a grip. Beginners can use either assisted pull-up machines or resistance bands while trying to master this exercise.

- **Chin-ups:** This is a variation of pull-ups, where your palms face you and the distance between the grips is shorter. It is easier as compared to pull-ups. Same technique, caution and repetitions need to be followed in this case also.

  Chin-ups differ from pull-ups when it comes to intensity and it hits different targeted muscles. In this exercise, the primarily impacted muscles are the biceps, while lats are also put to work to an extent.

- **Push-ups:** People boast about the number of push-ups they can do at a go. This exercise appears to be easy, but is more technical. It is mostly about the position of hands and palms, direction of elbows and the lowest your body can get. A well-postured push-up provides immense benefit. You can start with 30 push-ups in three sets, and then try to reach 45 to 60 per set, when comfortable.

  There is a wide variety of push-ups that targets different muscle groups—inclined, declined, weighted, wide-grip, narrow-grip, diamond-grip—to name a few. Push-ups make the shoulders, chest muscles and the triceps work.

- **Squats:** Squats do wonders if done properly. Ensure that your hip goes backward to allow your core to balance itself in a way that your body weight does not fall on your knees when you bend them. Else, it will hurt the knees. You should do these with your legs spaced wide in a comfortable position. Start with 30 squats, but try to reach 50 or 60 when comfortable.

Squat is a wonderful compound exercise; it works the quads, hams, glutes, calves and even the core. There are multiple variations of squats as well. The most common forms are done with a barbell on the back just below the neck. Pay attention to your form. There is a risk of injuring the muscles in your back, knee and spine. The most important tip is to ensure that the knees do not protrude above the foot when you lower your body. Since heavy weights are commonly used, it is advisable to perform the exercise using a Smith machine rather than with barbells.

- **Plank:** A five-minute plank is very refreshing. Plank has many variations. You can start with an elbow plank, and then move to a one-leg raise being on your elbows. You can then raise each side of your body alternatively, being on one elbow and leg each time. You can end the plank with a hindu push-up or doing elbow plank again.

  Though mainly touted as the core exercise, plank is a wholesome compound exercise that also tones the shoulders, arms, leg muscles along with the core. If you are new to planks, it is better to start with 30 seconds planks and gradually increase the hold time.

Sample Exercises to Achieve a Particular Goal

There are millions of workout routines. Below is a sample exercise, which has to be accompanied with the right diet plan. General rule of thumb for everyone no matter what routine is followed:

1. Every body part should go through an intensive training at least once a week.
2. Adequate amount of protein, balance of carbs and healthy fats should be consumed.
3. For weight loss: Eat 500–800 kcal less than maintenance calories (healthy rate of weight loss of 2–2.5 kg per month).
4. For weight gain: Eat 500–800 kcal excess from maintenance calories (healthy rate of weight gain of 2–2.5 kg per month).

Weight Loss Exercises

Weight loss is just not to burn more calories by doing only cardiovascular exercises, but by doing a full body exercise accompanied with cardiovascular exercises to get better results. Here is a sample schedule for such a regime.

This is for six days a week. If you miss any day, continue the missed day exercise the next day. The rest day should be a complete rest day, but keep the diet in check and do normal body movements.

Day 1: 75-minutes workout

5 minutes of stretches: Knee, ankle, neck, biceps, shoulder and triceps and some push-ups

5 minutes of plank: 1 minute elbow plank, 1 minute side plank (both sides), 1 minute each leg raise plank; increase the duration with practice

3 sets of abdominal crunches with folded legs: 20 repetitions each

3 sets of leg raises, 15 repetitions each

3 sets of body weight squats

5 minutes of stretches: ankles, knees, shoulders, biceps and triceps to end the routine

Day 2: 75-minutes workout

5 minutes of stretches
30 minutes of treadmill (jogging or brisk walking) or cycling or cross trainer, on a daily rotation basis
5 minutes of plank
3 sets of abdominal crunches, 20 repetitions each
3 sets of mountain climbing, 15 repetitions each
3 sets of body weight squats
5 minutes stretches to end the routine

Day 3: 75 minutes (Upper-body workout using light weights)

5 minutes of stretches
3 sets of normal or declined push-ups, 20 repetitions each
2 sets of Chin-ups, 10–15 repetitions each

Chest workouts (lightweight to normal weight, more repetitions)
Chest: Flat bench press 2 sets, 15–12 repetitions
Chest: 2 sets of inclined bench presses, 15–12 repetitions each

Chest: 2 sets of flat bench dumbbell flies, 15–12 repetitions each

Triceps: 2 sets of flat bench triceps extensions, 15–10 repetitions each
Triceps: 2 sets of cable push-downs, 15–10 repetitions
Triceps: 2 sets of back dips, 1–10 repetitions

Back: 2 sets of seated cable rows (close grip), 15–10 repetitions

Back: 2 sets of cable pull-down (wide grip), 15–10 repetitions
Back: 2 sets of bent over rows, 25–20 repetitions

Biceps: 2 sets of straight bar curls, 15–12 repetitions each
Biceps: 2 sets of preacher curls, 15–12 repetitions each
Biceps: 2 sets of concentration curls, 20–15 repetitions each
5 minutes of stretches to end the routine

Day 4: 75 minutes

5 minutes of stretches
30 minutes of treadmill (Jogging or brisk walking) or cycling or cross trainer, on a daily rotation basis
5 minutes of plank
3 sets of abdominal crunches, 20 repetitions each
3 sets of mountain climbing, 15 repetitions each
3 sets of body weight squats
5 minutes of stretches to end the routine

Day 5: 75 minutes

5 minutes of stretches
30 minutes of treadmill (jogging or brisk walking) or cycling or cross trainer, on a daily rotation basis
5 minutes of plank
3 sets of abdominal crunches, 25 repetitions each
3 sets of bicycle crunches, 25 repetitions each
3 sets of mason twist, 25 repetitions 3 times
5 minutes of stretches to end the routine

Day 6: 75 minutes

5 minutes of stretches
2 sets of squats, 20 repetitions each
3 sets of leg extensions, 15–10 repetitions each (increasing

weights in each set, with less repetitions)
3 sets of bar squats or dumbbell squats, 15–10 repetitions each
3 sets of hack squats, 15–10 repetitions each
3 sets of leg presses, 15–10 repetitions each
4 sets of leg curls, 15–10 repetitions each
3 sets of straight leg dead lifts, 15–10 repetitions each
3 sets of lunges with dumbbells, 15–10 repetitions each
3 sets of seated calf raises, 25–15 repetitions each
3 sets of standing calf raises, 25–15 repetitions each
5 minutes of stretches to end the routine

Day 7: Full rest day

After 7–8 weeks, you can add more variation to abdominal crunches, lower abdominal workout and increase the repetitions.

Weight Gain Exercises

Day 1: Chest, triceps and abs: 75 minutes

5 minutes: Knee stretch, biceps, triceps, shoulder stretches
3 sets of normal or declined push-ups, 20 repetitions each
2 sets of chin-ups, 10–15 repetitions each
2 sets of parallel bar dips, 10–15 repetitions each
Chest: 3 sets of flat bench presses, 15–8 repetitions each
Chest: 2 sets of inclined bench presses, 15–8 repetitions each
Chest: 3 sets of flat bench dumbbell flies, 15–8 repetitions each
Chest: 2 sets of cable cross over, 25 to 20 repetitions each

Triceps: 3 sets of flat bench triceps extentions, 15–10 repetitions each

Triceps: 3 sets of cable push-downs, 15–10 repetitions each
Triceps: 3 sets of back dips, 15–10 repetitions each
Triceps: 2 sets of diamond push-ups, 20–15 repetitions each

Abs: 3 sets of declined sit-ups, 25–15 repetitions each
Abs: 3 sets of cable crunches, 25–15 repetitions each
Abs: 3 sets of leg raises, 25–12 repetitions each
5–10 minutes stretches to end the routine

Day 2: Back, biceps and calves: 75 minutes

Stretches: 5 minutes
3 sets of normal or declined push-ups, 20 repetitions each
3 sets chin-ups, 10–15 repetitions each
2 sets parallel bar dips, 10–15 repetitions each

Back: 3 sets of seated cable rows (close grip), 15–10 repetitions each
Back: 3 sets of cable pull-downs (wide grip), 15–10 repetitions each
Back: 3 sets of cable pull-down (close grip), 15–10 repetitions each
Back: 3 sets of bent over rows, 25–20 repetitions each

Bicep: 3 sets of straight bar curls, 15–10 repetitions each
Bicep: 3 sets of preacher curls, 15–10 repetitions each
Bicep: 3 sets of dumbbell hammer curls, 15–10 repetitions each
Bicep: 2 sets of concentration curls, 20–15 repetitions each

Calves: 3 sets of seated calf raises, 25–15 repetitions each
Calves: 3 sets of standing calf raises, 25–15 repetitions each
5 minutes of stretches to end the routine

Day 3: 75 minutes generic workout

5 minutes of stretches and push-ups
30 minutes of treadmill (jogging or brisk walking) or cycling or cross trainer, on a daily rotation basis
5 minutes of plank (1 minute elbow, 1 minute each leg raise, 1 minute of each side raise)
3 sets of abdominal crunches, 25 repetitions each
3 sets of bicycle crunches, 25 repetitions each
3 sets of body weight squats

Day 4: Shoulder, traps and abs: 75 minutes

Stretches: 5 minutes

3 sets of normal or declined push-ups, 20 repetitions each
3 sets of chin-ups, 10–15 repetitions each
2 sets of parallel bar dips, 10–15 repetitions each

Shoulder: 3 sets of lateral dumbbell raises, 15–10 repetitions (increasing weights in each set, with less repetitions) each
Shoulder: 3 sets of front dumbbell raises, 15–10 repetitions each
Shoulder: 3 sets of rear deltoid raises, 15–10 repetitions each
Shoulder: 2 sets of car reverse pec deck, 15–10 repetitions each

Traps: 3 sets of straight bar shrugs, 15–10 repetitions each
Traps: 3–4 sets of dumbbell shrugs, 15–10 repetitions each

Abs: 3 sets of declined sit ups, 25–15 repetitions each
Abs: 3 sets of cable crunches, 25–15 repetitions each
Abs: 3 sets of leg raises, 25–15 repetitions each
5 minutes of stretches to end the routine

Day 5: Quadriceps, hamstrings and calves: 75 minutes

5 minutes of stretches
Body weight squats
Quadriceps: 3 sets of leg extensions, 15–10 repetitions (increasing weights in each set, with less repetitions) each

Quadriceps: 3 sets of bar squat or dumbbell squats, 15–10 repetitions each
Quadriceps: 3 sets of hack squats, 15–10 repetitions each
Quadriceps: 3 sets of leg press, 15–10 repetitions each

Hamstrings: 3 sets of leg curls, 15–10 repetitions each
Hamstrings: 3 sets of straight leg dead lift, 15–10 repetitions each
Hamstrings: 3 sets of lunges with dumbbells, 15–10 repetitions each

Calves: 3 sets of seated calf raises, 25–15 repetitions each
Calves: 3 sets of standing calf raises, 25–15 repetitions each
5 minutes of stretches to end the routine

Day 6: 75 minutes generic workout

Stretches and push-ups: 5 minutes

30 minutes of treadmill (jogging or brisk walking) or cycling or cross trainer, on a daily rotation basis
5 minutes of plank
3 set of abdominal crunches, keeping the leg perpendicular to the body, 25 repetitions each
3 sets of burpees, 10 repetitions each
3 sets of body weight squats
5 minutes of stretches to end the routine

Endurance and Stamina

Have you heard of marathon, triathlon, ironman or fit man competitions? They are all required to have an excellent stamina and extra ordinary endurance.

We have talked a lot about endurance. Let's now talk about what these exercises actually comprise of? It increases the strength and stamina, helps to lose weight, makes your body slim and athletic.

Traditional weight lifting when clubbed with various endurance exercises too give better results. These days, gyms advertise High Intensity Interval Training (HIIT), boot camp workouts, stepper workouts, tyre workouts, mix of strength and cardio as a part of functional training workouts.

Here is a list of some HIIT workouts that help to build the endurance:

- Burpees
- Plank hold (different types)
- Mountain climbing
- Squats
- Squat jumps
- Knee tuck jumps
- High knee jumps and many more

Endurance training is programmed in such a way that there should be around 30-seconds gap between sets and between different exercises to enable better results.

Reducing the Paunch and the Myth of Six-packs

If there is one body part that speaks volumes about a person's fitness, it is definitely the midsection. Just a casual look at someone's waistline says a lot about the individual's condition. A chiseled core not only screams about the owner's commitment, discipline and lifestyle, but is also a valuable asset that is often revered and proudly flaunted as 'six-packs'. Aesthetics aside, a toned and strong core is a critical component that comes handy in daily activities at home, office or elsewhere.

The six-packs rage

Over the past couple of decades, six-pack abs has become very popular. Bollywood is a major source of this popularity. Washboard abs are a treat to the eyes; it makes a person look fit. A narrow waistline and a proportionate body is a fair indicator of one's good health.

There is no dearth of free advices when it comes to this favorite topic and everyone has their own take on it:

*'Do hundred crunches a day, your tummy will be gone soon.'

'Drink hot lemon tea with honey first thing in the morning, and it melts your tummy.'

*'My coach has given an exercise to convert stomach fat into ab muscles.'

*'Use the slimming belt.'

*'I am going to lose fat just from my tummy.'

'Run 5 kms on an empty stomach in the morning.'

Some of the above advices do help, and some are plain bad (those which are marked with an asterisk).

Let us go back to our childhood and reflect how your belly looked and why it has changed since then. The answer is simple that you consume more calories than what your body needs.

When you were younger, you were active, indulged in sports, walked/cycled/took the bus to travel, etc. Your body was growing, and it needed more fuel. So, even if you ate junk food occasionally, it did not pose to be a problem. Now, you are not as active. You have a job; you drive to work and attend weekend parties. You don't partake in any kind of sports and fill yourself to the brim with late night snacks while watching TV, at office-sponsored buffet lunches and the list goes on. A 30-minutes walk is not enough to burn extra calories. Therefore, the mid-section of your body starts to bulge.

So how can you go get a flat tummy?

A simple answer is to reduce the calorie intake to a level that is lower than what your body needs for the maintenance and allow the stored fat to burn.

It is better to lose weight at a moderate pace than to indulge in extreme measures. Loss of 1.5–2 kgs per month is believed to be a healthy rate. This calls for a caloric deficit of 500–700 calories per day.

What does this mean?

Your body needs 2,000 calories per day to perform regular activities and the target is to create a 500-calorie deficit. You could do the following:

Option A: Eat 1,500 calories; no exercise is necessary.
Option B: Eat 1,700 calories and burn 200 calories by running, strength training, etc.
Option C: Eat 2,000 calories and burn 500 calories.

Option B definitely looks reasonable, where you do not need to starve or over exert to burn off a ton of calories. Moreover, the moderate activity you do to burn 200 calories is good for the heart and cardiovascular health.

You must have noticed that a fair bit of math is involved. You need to learn the caloric value of every bit of food you consume throughout the day and plan accordingly. There is a lot of information available online related to the daily caloric requirement calculator for a person based on their age, weight and height. There are calculators that tell your body the fat percentage, caloric value of every type of food, etc.

If you are unable to lose weight over a long time, you are obviously eating too much and/or exercising too less.

Weight Loss vs Fat Loss

Before we get into details of weight loss, let's bust a popular myth—spot reduction is impossible.

If you want to lose that bulging gut, the whole body weight needs to be reduced. This is something like formatting the hard disc drive of your computer when it gets infected with a stubborn virus. Spot reductions are only possible through cosmetic surgery, and let's not get into that!

Weight loss and fat loss are different. Weight loss is the result seen in a person after he or she has shed the surplus weight. Just ensure that you burn more than you consume, you will be guaranteed of weight loss.

Fat loss is similar to weight loss, but it also includes maintaining and toning the muscle. While it is not possible to direct the body to burn only fat, ensure to preserve muscle by making the groups of muscles workout regularly and consume enough protein. This will give you a toned and athletic body.

Body Fat Percentage and the Paunch

A bulging belly is an indication of a very high body fat percentage. Typically, men with more than 25 per cent of body fat will have protruding bellies, and the motive should be to bring it down to manageable levels:

1. Body fat brought down to 17–20 per cent result in disappearance of the bulge.
2. Whereas, body fat lowered to 14–17 per cent will bring a visibly pleasing flat core.
3. Anything lesser than these, you show the first signs of the much adored six-packs. This will be clearly visible when the body fat percentage drops down to single digits.

The Core Workout

There are tons of core exercises, many touted as 'the holy grail' for chiseled washboard abs. In fact, all these exercises tone the core muscles making them stronger. However, no matter how much you make your core work, its effect will only show when the layer of fat is burnt out in the mid-section. Working the core does not burn tummy fat. Many people do not work the core separately since it gets indirectly impacted during compound exercises like squats. There are detailed exercises per body part in this book, but if you want to know the bare minimum set, plain old crunches, leg raises, planks and mountain climbs are some of the good ones.

> **Caution** Your paunch can return in a few months if a balanced diet and exercise is not maintained.

Every person who has an acquaintance with fitness knows how treacherous the journey towards a flat tummy is. It takes tremendous courage and sacrifice to learn to start saying 'no' and to pass on that delicious chicken biriyani and the dessert that follows it. Often it comes to a point when you start to question the whole point of fitness and cannot even eat what you love. To have a chiseled core is not a destination but a continuous journey. You have to eat clean, exercise regularly and avoid binging on food or drinks. A couple of months of mindless gluttony is all it takes to nullify years of hard work; it is both sad and painful. The good news is that there is no permanent damage and the body is a wonderful machine that can be tweaked and tuned as long as there is a will to do so!

> **Caution** There is no relation between the dietary fat and the fat stored in our body. In fact, any excess food (carbohydrates, protein or fats) is converted into fat by the body. Fats should be an essential part of the diet for the body to function properly. Healthy fats can be found in the form of flax seeds/oils, fish oils, nuts, seeds, etc.

Fat and muscles are different kind of tissues that can either be lost or gained, but never 'converted' to/from each other. Generally, loss of fat layers result in exposing the muscles underneath, giving a perception that fat has turned to muscle.

SPECIAL SECTION #2

Fitness through Running

ASH NATH

8-time Boston Qualifier, the fastest Indian at the Comrade Ultra Marathon and the thrice winner at the Mumbai Marathon veteran category.

Why Running

It is probably the most popular fitness activity worldwide and provides an incredible feeling of achievement. To become a runner is easy with no membership fee and little equipment needed. Just lace up and you are good to go. The tricky part here is to stay a runner and keep reminding yourself that millions have done it before you.

In the running skills workshops that I host across India, the profile of participants range from 18-year-old youngsters to senior citizens, as everyone is now recognizing the merits of fitness. Many had hesitated in the beginning but very soon were hooked by the runner's high.

The sheer decision to adopt running makes you a winner and you enjoy a healthier lifestyle, witness wonderful scenery, meet fascinating individuals and revel in the new you.

Simple Common Sense

While running welcomes everyone, it would be prudent to get the following done before jumping into any training regime:

- **Basic Health Check-up:** Visit any decent clinic and get a medical check-up, inclusive of blood test and body composition. Awareness about your vitamin-D and B-12, haemoglobin, blood pressure, blood sugar and cholesterol levels are important. And, if you have led a largely sedentary life, then an Exercise ECG would be advisable too.

  If any of the results are outside the normal limits, do consult your physician and/or dietician. Usually, addressing 'gaps' in your diet will cater to any shortcomings; however, supplementation may be necessary.

- **Resting and Normal Heart Rate:** When you wake up, measure your pulse rate using a simple second's watch while still in bed. This establishes your Resting Heart Rate. Later in the day, do the same to establish your Normal Heart Rate. Both these should show a downward trend as your fitness improves.

  Maintain a health folder and enter the above data as Control Group to serve as a reference point to assess your improvement as you repeat the tests periodically.

- **Proper Running Form:** Invest the time to get your running form evaluated by an expert. Visit http://catalystsports.in/Scheduling.php for guidance. Improper technique will give suboptimal results for all your training efforts, and could result in an injury.

How To Go about Your Training

Avoid the mindset of 'More is Better' and 'No Pain, No Gain' that most beginners adopt. Instead, start slow and adhere to gradual progression of increasing the levels of stress over time, as that will minimize the likelihood of injuries. Consult a dietician to ensure your nutrition requirements are streamlined and supports your training efforts for better results.

Target to train at least 5 days weekly, 60–90 minutes on weekdays and slightly longer on weekends, with each session comprising of a warm up, main workout/s and a cool down. Remind yourself that success happens from consistency and moderate exercise done regularly pays greater dividends than strenuous exercise done intermittently.

Don't immediately jump into structured training but ease yourself into a programme, as follows:

Phase One (3-6 months depending on your present fitness level)

Goal is to improve overall fitness and so Strength-Flexibility-Core are priority hard workouts done across three days with supporting easy cardio workouts like jogging, cycling, swimming, elliptical and rowing across two days.

With respect to running, opt for easy jogging, even brisk walks, till the body gets stronger to handle greater impact forces. Follow the 'talk test' as a guide to assess if you are running too fast. If you can't talk in complete sentences while running, you are running too fast. Occasional classes of yoga, Zumba, Pilates, aerobics and spinning are welcome, as they add variety to training and keeps interest levels high.

Remember to update your fitness folder by tracking weekly your heart rate, your body composition monthly and record your blood test results quarterly. Women runners should pay attention to their iron levels.

Phase Two (1-3 months)

Add an extra training day (so 5 days becomes 6 now) as fitness improves, and allocate this extra day to an additional cardio workout.

Shift emphasis and now make cardio your priority hard-workout, with Strength-Flexibility-Core as your easy days-workout. Here, 'hard' implies increasing either intensity or the time/distance of cardio workouts from that followed in Phase One.

Continue to update your fitness folder.

Phase Three (Ongoing)

By this stage, you should be feeling like a different person altogether, and this would be supported by an improved heart rate, body composition and blood tests results, besides visibly greater strength and cardio levels.

Continue with a 6-day training routine, but now add yet another day for cardio (3 days becomes 4 now) and reduced Strength-Flexibility-Core workouts (3 days becomes 2 now).

There are principally four forms of running workouts—speed, tempo, endurance and recovery runs—that manifests in your training plan, with an occasional hill run.

Pre-training Check List

Ask yourself these simple quick questions:

- Am I willing to sacrifice most weekends for 2-3 months?
- Is my family/partner supportive of my passion?
- Is my professional life relatively light across the coming months?
- Is my diet balance and healthy?
- Am I largely injury free?
- Am I free from any major health issues?

Only if your answers to the questions above are 'yes', should you start training for a race.

Way Forward

Ideally, you should enroll yourself in a running event as this will give you a goal and act as a strong motivator in your training. The thought of 'racing' may initially bring out a sweat but taking part in running events is actually a good decision no matter how you finally perform. The excitement of the race, the camaraderie between runners and your own sense of personal triumph will stay forever in your memory. Don't be surprised if you find yourself hooked and become a regular participant in running events.

Choosing a Running Event

There is no dearth of races nowadays, but you should be clear about your motives when choosing the right one to ensure a good running experience.

Larger events have thousands of runners so there will always be a group running at your pace. Add the media coverage, large crowd support, better facilities and you will literally have a grand party. The drawbacks are that there is a lack of personal touch, the course is crowded and you need to report several hours prior to the actual race. The registration fee is likely on the higher side as well.

Smaller events are quite the reverse with personal attention given to runners and you can report a few minutes prior to the start. You waste no time in parking, holding area and pushing through the crowd of runners in the race. What's beneficial is that you are likely to find an event more conveniently located to your residence.

Frankly, if the timing of a race is important for you, a smaller event is the smarter choice, whereas, if a memorable experience is your motive then a larger race will suit you better.

Choosing Your Run Distance

Progress smartly and build your running experience by initially doing shorter race distances like the 5 km and 10 km. This experience will hold you in good stead, as you will strengthen your musculo-skeletal system and become a stronger runner.

While many runners opt for half and full marathons, it is perfectly fine to focus on the shorter distances if that is where your interest lies and suits your schedule. As you go forth in this journey, you will discover where your passion lies and remember to not get influenced by others. Fitness is determined not by the sheer mileage, but by smartly training with some variety and consistency, accompanied by good eating habits.

Training Guidelines

- Hard/Easy
  - Alternate hard with easy training, within a week and across weeks.
- Window of Opportunity
  - Kick-start recovery by consuming 4:1 ratio of carb: protein within 30

minutes of completing a workout.
- Protein supplementation is advisable, especially for vegetarians and vegans.
- Running Shoes
  - Have 2-3 pairs and alternate between them.
  - Lighter shoes for shorter, more cushioned shoes for longer runs.
- Hydration
  - Stay hydrated. Use the 'pee test' where pale yellow is healthy.
- Fueling
  - Water is fine for workouts lasting up to an hour. Energy drinks for longer workouts.
- Sleep
  - Ensure 7-9 hours of sleep. A nap during the day is good.

Common Race Distances

5-10 km:

This is the most beginner-friendly distance as it is challenging but is also a realistic distance that can be accomplished through a mix of moderate fitness and training, and build a strong foundation to attempt longer distances.

Half marathon (21.1 km):

You need to commit to training well for a half marathon, but can justifiably call yourself a long-distance runner. It is long enough to challenge yourself, at the same time short enough to run fairly fast. Through good time management, you can comfortably train for it without making major adjustments in your life.

Marathon (42.2 km):

The marathon is viewed with equal degree of awe and fear as no matter how much you may have prepared, it will still test your mental and physical limits. Before you take the plunge, be clear about your motivations, otherwise the hours and months of disciplined training will have you question your purpose.

PACES FOR SPEED WORKOUTS BASED ON 5-KM TIME TRIAL							
HYPOTHETICAL EXAMPLE	TIME TAKEN FOR 5-KM	HYPOTHETICAL TIME OF 25 MINUTES*					
	TIME IN SECS/400M LOOPS	25X60/12.5** = 120 SECS OR 2 MINUTES PER 400M					
	200M	400M	800M	1000M	1200M	1600M	2000M
NO. OF INTERVALS	8 TO 16	8 TO 12	5 TO 6	4 TO 6	3 TO 4	3 TO 4	2 TO 3
400M PACE*** (REFER TO INDEX)	108 SECS (1.48)	110 SECS (1.50)	112 SECS (1.52)	113 SECS (1.53)	115 SECS (1.55)	156 SECS (1.56)	117 SECS (1.57)
ACTUAL TIME PER INTERVAL	54 SECS (0.54)	110 SECS (1.50)	224 SECS (3.44)	283 SECS (4.43)	345 SECS (5.45)	464 SECS (7.44)	585 SECS (9.45)
RECOVERY TIME BETWEEN INTERVALS	60 SECS	90 SECS	SAME AS INTERVAL TIME	UPTO 80% OF INTERVAL TIME	UPTO 70% OF INTERVAL TIME	UPTO 60% OF INTERVAL TIME	UPTO 50% OF INTERVAL TIME
INDEX							
*	HYPOTHETICAL TIME FOR 5KM. INPUT YOUR OWN ACTUAL 5KM TIME TRIAL						
**	5KM (OR 5000M) IMPLIES 12.5 LAPS OF 400M						
***	TO DEDUCT X-SECONDS FROM 400M–5KM TIME (TAKEN AS 120 SECS HERE)						
200M	DEDUCT 12 SECS. 120 - 12 = 108 SECS SO 54 PER 200M (OR 0.54 MINUTE)						
400M	DEDUCT 10 SECS. 120 - 10 = 110 SECS PER 400M (OR 1.50 MINUTE)						
800M	DEDUCT 8 SECS. 120 - 8 = 112 SECS SO 224 PER 800M (OR 3.44 MINUTES)						
1000M	DEDUCT 7 SECS. 120 - 7 = 113 SECS SO 283 PER 1000M (OR 4.43 MINUTES)						
1200M	DEDUCT 5 SECS. 120 - 5 = 115 SECS SO 345 PER 1200M (OR 5.45 MINUTES)						
1600M	DEDUCT 4 SECS. 120 - 4 = 116 SECS SO 464 PER 1600M (OR 7.44 MINUTES)						
2000M	DEDUCT 3 SECS. 120 - 3 = 117 SECS SO 585 PER 2000M (OR 9.45 MINUTES)						

Note: A hypothetical time of 25 minutes was taken for the 5 km time trial to arrive at the stipulated paces from 200 m to 2,000 m speed intervals. Periodically, say 4–6 weeks, the time trial should be repeated as improved fitness should reflect in a faster timing and a fresh calculation for speed intervals should be done using that lesser time.

PACES FOR TEMPO RUN WORKOUTS BASED ON 5-KM TIME TRIAL			
HYPOTHETICAL EXAMPLE	TIME TAKEN FOR 5 KM	HYPOTHETICAL TIME OF 25 MINUTES*	
	TIME PER KM	25X60 SECS/5 = 300 SECS OR 5.00 KM	
IF TRAINING FOR ...	5 - 10 KM	HALF MARATHON	MARATHON
DISTANCE PER SET	3 KM	5 KM	6 KM
NO. OF SETS	2 TO 3		
PER KM PACE BASIS 5 KM TIME TRIAL, IN MINUTES	5.00	5.00	5.00
TEMPO PACE PER KM, IN MINUTES	ADD 10 SECS	ADD 15 SECS	ADD 20 SECS
	5.10	5.15	5.20
TIME PER SET IN MINUTES	15.30	26.15	32.00
RECOVERY TIME BETWEEN INTERVALS	3 MINUTES	2 MINUTES	90 SECS

Note: Using the same hypothetical example of 25 minutes time trial reflects a 5.00-km pace. Naturally as the distance increases, the pace/km will fall off and hence the buffer per km reflected in the tempo pace per set.

PACES FOR LONG RUNS BASED ON 5 KM TIME TRIAL				
HYPOTHETICAL EXAMPLE	TIME TAKEN FOR 5 KM		HYPOTHETICAL TIME OF 25 MINUTES*	
	TIME PER KM		25X60 SECS/5 = 300 SECS OR 5.00 KM	
IF TRAINING FOR ...	5 KM	10 KM	HALF MARATHON	MARATHON
LONG RUNS IN KMS	6	13	24	32
PER KM PACE BASIS 5 KM TIME TRIAL, IN MINUTES	5.00	5.00	5.00	5.00
LONG RUN ADJUSTED PACE PER KM	ADD 15 SECS	ADD 20 SECS	ADD 45 SECS	ADD 60 SECS
	5.15 KM	5.20 KM	5.45 KM	6.00 KM
TIME TAKEN FOR LONG RUNS, IN MINUTES (HRS)	31.30	69.20 (1.09.20)	138 (2.18.00)	192 (3.12.00)

DRINKS BREAK	NIL	NIL	INTERMITTENT SHORT BREAKS FOR FUELING AND HYDRATION. CONSIDER EVERY 5-6 KM

NOTE: Long runs may be done continuously, as is usually the case for 5 and 10 km runners given the modest distance, or with intermittent fueling and hydration breaks. Some distance runners prefer to drink on-the-move while others choose to stop and refresh.

Workout Sessions (refer to grid to calculate paces)

Long runs: Much like the little black dress every woman must have, the long run is the bedrock of any training plan. You may have all the speed in the world but if you lack endurance, you will simply not finish your race.

5 km: Start with a mix of walk-jog-walk until you can comfortably jog 4-6 km at a stretch. Then do this once a week.

10 km: Gradually scale up from doing 6-8 km to 10 km until you can manage to run 13 km at a stretch. Then, do this distance every fortnight till your race. Besides improving your cardiovascular ability, the knowledge that you have run further during trainings makes the actual race seem easier.

Half marathon: If you take up one of these weekly, your approach to the long runs will vary depending on whether you are skewed towards speed/fast twitch or endurance/slow twitch muscle fibre.

In the former case, you should scale up cautiously doing 16-18 km to 20 km long runs while maintaining a constant speed. In the latter case, you can scale up faster and go longer doing 16-18 km to 20-24 km long runs at lower speeds.

Marathon: The maximum distance you should do in training is 32 km. The benefits of running any further are not worth the wear and tear, which will delay recovery and affect future training. Remind yourself that on the race day, you will have tapered, carbo-loaded and will be able to depend on the excitement factor to give you the energy to run further.

Build up your weekly long runs gradually, 24-27-30-32 km with every third week as a rest week.

Speed runs: The knowledge that you can run fast is a confidence booster and allows you to surge past others when needed.

5 km: A sheer speed is critical given the modest distance. Therefore, focus on short and medium intervals of 200-400 m to 800-1,000 m, twice weekly.

10 km: A fine balance of speed and endurance is needed; so focus on medium and long intervals of 1,000-1,200 m to 1,600-2,000 m, once weekly.

Half Marathon: This is similar to the 10 km speed run, but requires greater muscular endurance given the longer distance. Focus on the same medium and long intervals distances, but increase the number of repetitions in a workout. Once a week is sufficient.

Marathon: While endurance is the key given that the primary challenge is the sheer distance, speed workouts help make the slower marathon pace seem much easier. So, focus on long intervals of 1,000-2,000 m, but reduce the overall frequency of your speed workouts. Once in a week or even in a fortnight is fine.

Tempo runs: The capability to hold a steady pace for a long duration comes from doing tempo runs in training.

5 and 10 km: Two or three sets of 3 km with a three-minute recovery jog, twice weekly.

Half marathon: Two or three sets of 4-5 km with a two-minute recovery jog, once weekly.

Marathon: Two or three sets of 6-8 km with 90 seconds recovery jog, once weekly.

Recovery runs: As their namesake, these are slow and easy runs, which serve as active recovery to allow your body to bounce back.

5 and 10 km: Only needed during training when the intensity levels are high and then once a week.

Half marathon: Budget for one recovery run each week.

Marathon: Besides their active recovery benefit, these also add mileage to your weekly plan, which contributes to the total time spent on your feet. Budget two such runs per week.

Supplemental workouts: These include cross training, strength training and core-cum-flexibility workouts that boost your running performance and help minimize the likelihood of injuries. In phase three, these fit into the training plan as 'easy' workouts between hard run days.

Calculating the Paces for Your Run Workouts in Phase Three

Step 1: After a proper warm up, do a 5 km time trial on best effort basis on a largely flat terrain. Track would be ideal.

Note: If you are unable to run 5 km at a stretch, you can opt to run 3 × 1,600 m with a one-minute recovery break between attempts. Average the time for the three 1,600 m repeats, multiply this by 0.62 and add 9 seconds to arrive at your predicted 5 km race pace.

Step 2: Go to pace charts (speed/tempo/long run) and factor in your 5 km race pace to arrive at your training paces.

Note: Periodically, repeat the 5 km time trial, say once monthly, as your fitness will have improved and repeat Step 2.

Step 3: Refer to 'workout sessions' and craft a weekly and monthly plan that is practical for yourself, basis your race distance and factors in your responsibilities in life.

Step 4: Start training!

Race Strategy

Most runners start too fast and burn out soon. Some run so conservatively that they begin to feel there is no fuel left. While a largely even pace with a faster finish section is ideal, novice runners should approach their race somewhat differently.

5 km: The modest distance implies you cannot play too conservative. So establish a comfortable rhythm until about 3 km when you dig deep to run faster till the end.

10 km: This requires managing energies better. Run steady till you cross the halfway mark. Run faster with the realization that the end isn't far.

Half Marathon: The objective should be to finish in a respectable time. So run steady until about 16 km, always feeling you are within your capabilities, after which you dig deep to hold the pace or even increase until the end.

Marathon: The objective should be to complete the distance without being intimidated by it. Target the 32 km mark in a relatively good state after which you can grit it out to the end.

Smart Advice

- *Scaling up:* Scale up (from 5 km to 10 km, 10 km to half marathon, and half to the full marathon) when you have finished the earlier distance a few times comfortably, and are ready to put in the necessary (longer) training for the next distance.
- *Keeping injuries at bay:* Most of the injuries from running revolve around issues that concern the joints and/or strained muscles, but these are not vocational hazards. With a smart approach to your training, you can avoid or, at least, minimize them. Injuries happen due to several reasons, namely:
  - Repetitive movement: Play it smart and include some cross-training to your routine.

- Insufficient strength/flexibility: Ensure that you are working on these aspects alongside your running workouts. Budget for an occasional massage session as a preventive measure
- Too much, too soon: Listen to your body and add greater stress only when you feel truly ready.

▶ *Maintaining fitness:* Remember that while your cardio fitness takes long to develop, you will lose it much faster if there is a long period of lay off. But the heart is just a muscle that requires some kind of workout like running or any other cardio fitness activity. Advice is to stay active.

Staying Motivated

Running is quite the social sport nowadays as most runners have regular jobs and yet find the time to follow their passion. While some may find the resolve within themselves to stay motivated, other short cuts serve equally well.

▶ *Run with a friend or a running group*: Having a partner/s increases the likelihood to adhere to your training regime. To know that someone is going to pick you up or wait for you at the park is a powerful motivator to get you out of the bed. Remind yourself that the distance is easier to cover when you share it with someone.

▶ *Run in nature*: While road is a commonplace to run, make it a point to occasionally run in the park and soak in the scenery.

▶ *Make music your companion*: This is especially useful for the longer runs, and on days when you feel low.

▶ *Get active online and share your experiences*: Running is a hot topic and you can find running forums online that share experiences and encourage each other.

▶ *Cross train*: Too much of anything can get tiresome so occasionally mix it up by joining a class of aqua jogging, aerobics, Zumba, TRX, cross fit and so forth. You will rediscover your mojo after running and return as a stronger refreshed person.

- *Adopt a cause*: A strong motivator is running for something larger than yourself. Many good causes seek support and you could help raise awareness/funds/support for them. The knowledge that your running is helping others will keep you going through rough patches.

Always maintain a balanced perspective and remember that running should enrich your life, not bog it down. There will be periods when you should devote your complete focus on the activity for best results. However, these periods must be interspersed with others when you allow yourself both mental and physical relief.

Always remember to play the long game and not get burnt out.

SPECIAL SECTION #3

Fitness through Yoga

LUVENA RANGEL
with contributions from
Pradeep Gowda, Director, a1000yoga Academy

In everyday life, most of us are well versed with the toll of the daily grind. The inevitable stress that we go through seems to be compounded for those professionals who constantly struggle to meet deadlines, deliver high impact and effective presentations, and at the end of the day, attempt to maintain a balanced social and personal life full of joy, happiness and good health. These activities and aspirations seem simple enough, yet, for most of us they also prove to be a daunting task; the result of which is consistently moving further away from reach.

It is common to find most professionals and executives struggling to find and maintain this balance. Fitness options, however, are a common workplace benefit offered currently to employees across sectors. Fitness has often been equated with constant effort—to maintain the body through 'working out'. The effort is usually justified by sweat, burn and pain—the core input to the result of a lean, toned body and perhaps a rush of adrenaline and endorphins. It works. We acknowledge that the result-oriented approach is useful and significantly effective. However, as a yoga practitioner, a yogi, let's just say, our goal is slightly different, the result a little refined, including elements that otherwise underplay our human-ness. Fitness, to a yogi, is a more compound experience, where all components of body, mind and spirit are balanced and in harmony.

In my observation, a consistent yoga practice has been a fundamental aspect of thriving and successful professionals. We have observed subtle as well as unmistakable changes in the behaviour and well-being quotient of a number of executives who have made a simple choice—showing up on the mat. Just showing up for a simple, yet consistent yoga practice has proven to be the only factor that has helped individuals build their power of concentration, cognition, motor skills as well as inter-personal relationships. The physical activity of yoga is a natural and gentle means to decongest the body after many hours of sitting in meetings, driving through traffic or simply straining oneself in front of the computer.

Asanas are postures that have qualitative benefits that accumulate with regular practice and show up as natural qualities in the personality of the practitioner. Specific series of postures generally have the inherent qualities of grounding, enhancing confidence, encouraging introspection, determination, focus, concentration, creativity, self-worth, steadfastness and other distinctive traits and a well-balanced class taps into all these possibilities just with a few moments of asana practice.

While the asanas by themselves are physical practices that stimulate and encourage movement, a core aspect of a complete yoga practice also includes conscious breathing and taking a few moments to calm the mind. One cannot stress enough about the importance of these two aspects for almost any individual, but for a professional, constantly surrounded by stressful triggers, some simple techniques can help bring about a state of balance even in the most infringing situations.

Pranayama practices are simple yet potent techniques that utilize the power of breath and prana to induce various states of emotional as well as behavioural changes. We have all experienced the short and exasperated breaths in a stressful situation—an angry client, a confrontational boss demanding a deadline submission or the frustration of making time for the family after a long and challenging week at the office. Breathing is a constant guideline to our emotional and physical state of being. Through pranayama, we can simply, yet powerfully, control our breathing to bring in a variety of experiences and qualities.

Starting the Day

Even under time crunch, two rounds of Surya Namaskar (Sun Salutation) can be incorporated into a daily regime for a total body workout without taking more than a few minutes. However, even the regularity of simply waking up and performing simple joint releasing movements, like pavan muktasan, neck or wrist rotations/gentle mobilization, and beginning the day with 5 to 10 minutes of body stillness—simply sitting still and observing the inflow and outflow of one's breath is a premise to begin the day on a positive note. Note that these morning practices, especially Surya Namaskar are ideally done on an empty stomach or with a gap of at least two hours after a breakfast and four hours after lunch.

A few common complaints that we hear of are listed below, along with some postures that may help to alleviate the symptoms (see Infograph at the end of this section):

Note: Allow ample time for food to be digested before these practices—at least two hours after breakfast and four hours after lunch.

General Well-being

As a way of life, yoga had originally been designed as a practice for general well-being. Our lifestyle has created the obstacles like poor or insufficient fitness, diseases and disorders. At the very least, a disciplined effort to include regular and focused mobility is one of the best ways to ensure that the body and all its parts are kept in good condition. The humble Surya Namaskara, although not a classical asana, is a series of postures that is a brilliant inclusion for overall wellness. It can be performed slowly as a warmup, faster for cardio training and in repetition for endurance and vigour. Even if one includes five sun salutes in a daily regime, it gives a brilliant start to physical as well as physiological suppleness.

To De-stress

Yogic or abdominal breathing is a technique where you inhale deeply to the count of five and exhale to the count of five. When you inhale, breathe in through your chest into the abdomen. Push out the air by tightening the abdominal muscles through the lungs from your nose.

Spine and Postural Management

A yoga practitioner should avoid compromising with the posture and spinal alignment. This is done to mobilize the spine in various directions through stretches and twists. Yoga, especially when performed under the guidance of a teacher, would help the practitioner find the right alignment in any asana. However, basic postures can be corrected by practising simple asanas like Tadasana (mountain pose) and by constantly being aware of the entire body during each asana. Proper posture would also help in alleviating knee and hip pain often caused due to improper spinal alignment and poor posture. This takes practice, but one would be surprised at how easily this progresses.

Neck and Back Problems

One of the most common complaints at workplace is neck and back strain and pain and most physicians will directly identify this as a postural symptom. Simple stretches that periodically mobilize the spine in different directions help to relax the tightened muscles and give respite to the body that is inching towards fatigue. The stretches are simple and easy to perform anywhere and at any time of the day. (See section 2 of the infograph below)

Loosening the joints and mobilizing the spine are simple yet effective practices for a healthy nervous system. Subsequently, a healthy nervous system means improved motor and cognitive skills that are crucial at workplace. It is better to be a relaxed and creative professional than a fatigued one with low creativity and drive.

Lower Back Pain

Bhujangasana (Cobra Pose) is ideal for lower back stiffness and pain. You may keep the feet slightly apart if necessary. Relax into the posture and hold for three to five deep breaths by paying attention to the lower back.

Shashankasana (Child's Pose) is a good relaxation pose and anyone can do it. However, if an individual is unable to completely bend forward, place a bolster or a cushion under the forehead or to support the arms. Knees can also be placed apart from each other if the abdomen needs to be accommodated. Breathe deeply and comfortably three to five times.

Neck Pain, Frozen Shoulder and Wrist Pain

The neck, shoulders and wrists are a complex constitution for this generation of people who are hooked onto laptops, computers, phones and other gadgets. A person's chronic predisposition to neck or shoulder aches due to the time spent looking at his or her phone is a widespread syndrome. However, apart from ergonomic changes, one can incorporate simple steps to relieve the problems of this professional hazard. Periodic neck, shoulder and wrist rotations (clockwise and anticlockwise) can help to keep these joints pain-free and will hardly take any time or space away from one's work station. As an added bonus, one can stand up to do these and take advantage of resting the spine from a prolonged seating position.

Lifestyle Diseases and Disorders

Poor lifestyle choices and a lot of stress has resulted in a number of lifestyle related diseases and disorders in our professional space. High blood pressure, diabetes, musculoskeletal disorders, obesity and infertility issues are all on the rise. Although yoga isn't a cure, we have observed a consistent improvement in the conditions from the practice of yoga.

Hatha Yoga has helped bring about a balance in our physiological imbalances without putting too much strain on our physical ability. Apart from encouraging the body towards regular mobility, the physical asanas have a direct influence on the organs and glands, whose malfunctioning is responsible for these conditions and disorders.

Weight Management

Obesity and weight management is a forerunner when it comes to lifestyle disorders today. While diet plays an important role, the influence of yoga matters when choosing the right form (Hatha or Ashtanga) to maximize the benefits of a weight management protocol. Both systems work in such a way that it boosts metabolism and tones the muscles in order to eliminate excess fat from the body. One might also consider certain asanas that would accelerate fat loss and body toning. Dhanurasana (Bow Pose), shalabhasana (Locust Pose), parsvakonasana (Side Angle Pose) and even trikonasana (Triangle Pose), if held for five and building up to eight deep breaths will help. The inclusion of twists like ardhamatsyendra will help in toning the oblique muscles.

Diabetes

Ardhamatsyendra (Sage Matsyendra's Pose) is a classical twist and a highly beneficial detoxifying posture, which cleanses and nourishes the organs in the abdominal region, especially the pancreas responsible for insulin and glucagon secretion. If the practitioner is unable to bring the arm across the opposite knee to twist, it is permissible to simply hold the knee and twist in the opposite direction. Maintain comfortable deep breathing for three to five times with a smile and relaxed shoulders.

Shavasana (Corpse Pose), the simple, yet highly potent posture allows the body to undergo conscious and deep relaxation. Today, diabetes has been largely called a lifestyle disorder due to the influence of stress. This asana allows the body to rest physically as well as mentally. Shavasana can be practised by itself or between asanas breathing deeply. Three to five deep breaths in Shavasana is ideal between asanas, but at the end of the practice, Shavasana can extend for a longer duration.

Blood Pressure

Gentle breathing and meditation along with a consistent but non-strenuous yoga practice is recommended for maintaining blood pressure. Specifically for hypertensive practitioners, they should avoid forward bends by bringing the head below the heart level and holding the breath in pranayama. During regular asana, care should be taken to encourage calm and regular breathing.

Thyroid Disorders and Metabolic Imbalances

Ustrasana (Camel Pose) should be avoided if you have knee injuries and inflammation. If it is difficult for you to reach for the toes in this pose, elevate the heels by bringing the toes closer to your fingers. In the final posture, relax your shoulders and breathe through your throat, holding the asanas for three to five deep breaths. This posture is also beneficial for the lower back pain.

Kandharasana (Bridge Pose) is an easily accessible asana that is highly beneficial for thyroid disorders, diabetes and back pain. Kandharasana helps to release muscular spasms in the lower back and is a posture of choice for chronic back pain due to improper posture as well as spinal health.

To Improve Concentration at Work

Bramari Pranayama is done by covering the ear flaps with the thumbs and resting the fingers on the crown of your head. Inhale deeply and hum while exhaling the breath feeling the vibrations in the head. This deeply soothing pranayama is highly beneficial in balancing the emotions after an emotional outburst, to build mental acuity and concentration before a test or an interview or that important business presentation.

Finally, simple meditative practices are easy to incorporate into everyday activities. Taking a break from any task and simply sitting with the eyes closed and consciously breathing is a highly revitalizing practice. Kaya Sthairyam, or body stillness, is a conscious application of gently coaching the mind to listen to your intention by requesting it to remain still and unmoving. The mind eventually follows this stillness and a state of meditative awareness is attained. One can practice this by sitting in a simple cross-legged Sukhasana posture or even on a chair, bench, against a wall or even while travelling.

To conclude, as a branch of living wisdom, yoga is a vast practice steeped in ancient wisdom, philosophy and culture—a tradition based on people and their desire to seek happiness and health. While fitness, today, may seem to come at a price, the purpose of yoga remains to bridge that gap between transaction and fulfilment. A transaction is something that aims to build wellness, good health and happiness, not just for the practitioner but also for the entire ecosystem—one that thrives on the overall growth and evolution of every individual component through peaceful harmony, mutual respect and co-existence. This practice is available to all of us as a means to experience these emotions and feelings, and let them into the society—our families, friends, colleagues and acquaintances.

SIMPLE DO-IT-YOURSELF
YOGA PRACTICE TO VITALIZE YOURSELF

- Choose a quiet, clutter-free space in any part of your home.
- Wear comfortable clothing.
- Do these on an empty stomach: Mornings after clearing bowels/ 2 hours after breakfast, 4 hours after lunch.
- If any health conditions, consult a physician.
- Optional: Take a shower before doing these practices to feel more supple and a sense of ease.

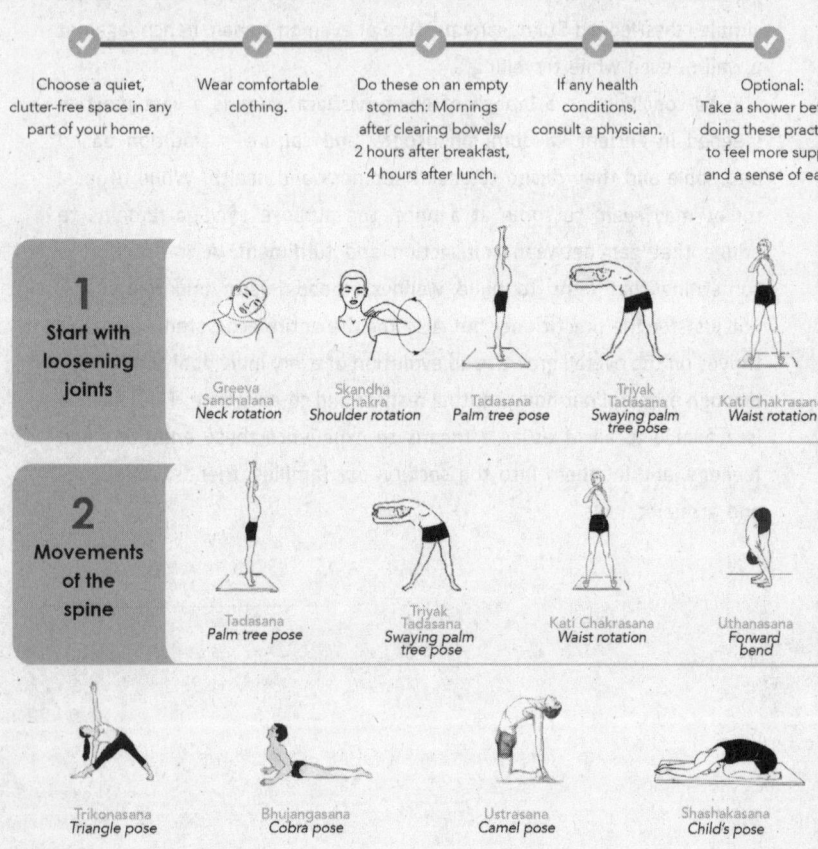

1 Start with loosening joints
- Greeva Sanchalana — Neck rotation
- Skandha Chakra — Shoulder rotation
- Tadasana — Palm tree pose
- Triyak Tadasana — Swaying palm tree pose
- Kati Chakrasana — Waist rotation

2 Movements of the spine
- Tadasana — Palm tree pose
- Triyak Tadasana — Swaying palm tree pose
- Kati Chakrasana — Waist rotation
- Uthanasana — Forward bend
- Trikonasana — Triangle pose
- Bhujangasana — Cobra pose
- Ustrasana — Camel pose
- Shashakasana — Child's pose

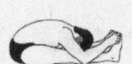
Pashchimottanasana
Seated Forward bend

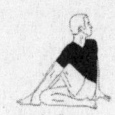
Ardh Matsyendrasana
Sage Matsyendra's pose

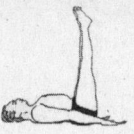
Uttanapadasana
Leg raises

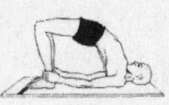
Kandharasana
Bridge pose

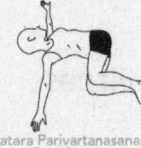
Jatara Parivartanasana
Spinal twist

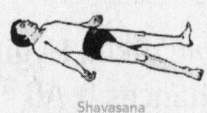
Shavasana
Corspe pose

3 Breath Awareness

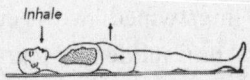

Yogic breathing or ratio and counting breaths
demonstration through abdominal breathing

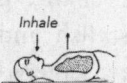

Yogic breathing
demonstration through chest breathing

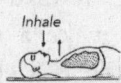

Yogic breathing
demonstration through collar bone breathing

4 Meditative practices

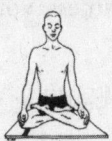
Kaya Sthairyam
Body stillness

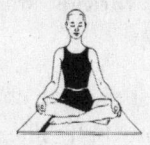
Sukhasana
Seated cross-legged pose

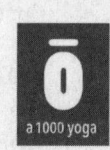
a 1000 yoga

www.a1000yoga.com

Fitness through Yoga

SIX

Style, Skin, Hygiene and Height: Fitness Enhances It All

The journey of fitness is intertwined with changes in personality. Such changes are not sudden but gradual. Let us consider how fitness enhances your style, impacts our skin and hygiene. We will also talk about the myth and reality of its impact on height in this beautiful journey.

You can reward yourself with the ever-changing wardrobe to make a right style statement. A stylish and well-fitted outfit is a clear indicator that you have entered the world of fitness. On a lighter note, it proves to be a very expensive reward as the wardrobe keeps changing according to various stages of fitness you keep achieving in this journey.

Style: The first sign of change in clothing you will notice is the size of your belt. The hole you used to fasten the belt to will seem to be too loose and the previous one too tight. I had to get a hole punched between the two. As most of my fat was deposited around my waist, it was a positive sign and this lifted my spirits and encouraged me to carry on.

My happiness did not last long as the new adjustment

of my belt was not permanent. Sometimes I needed to go back to the previous setting which left me puzzled. Rather than being disheartened, I tried to burn more calories by not using elevators in my office. I did not want to increase my cardio, which was anyway quite high, and more of it would result in tiredness, which would prevent me from doing other exercises well. Soon I realized that during such transitional times, these frequent fluctuations are normal and depending upon person, to person it takes time to stabilize.

On my next visit to the mall, I was tempted to try a pair of pants of size 36 instead of the one that measured 38. I wanted to try it when my wife was not around. When I found her busy in her section, I quickly moved to the men's section and picked up a size 36. My happiness knew no bounds. I came out of the fitting room and stood in front of the sales person. I was expecting some appreciation but he did not even notice my expression. I realized my foolishness and called him. He did not react and pulled out the measuring tape from his pocket to measure the length of the pants for alteration.

'No, I am asking, how is the fitting?' I was getting impatient.

'How do you feel? Is it comfortable?' He asked curiously.

I was puzzled and he quickly added, 'Breathe normally and see if it is not tight at your waist.'

I was going to shout at him for his rudeness, but then realized that I was taking short breaths and holding them too. I relaxed and he promptly responded.

'A little tight. Let me show you a few other brands, whose size 36 might fit you well.'

He brought a similar pair of trousers from the other

brand and it fitted me well. By then, my wife came looking for me.

'Look, I have reduced my waist. Size 36 is fitting me now.' I exclaimed to her.

'It is looking nice and hope you are comfortable too.' She smiled.

'I am,' I replied.

'I guess you shouldn't buy this.' she stated seriously.

'Why not?' I protested.

'It is simple. Your weight will fluctuate, and these pants could be tight for you again. It is better you wait for some more time.'

'That is why I asked him to try this other brand,' the salesperson jumped into the conversation much to my dismay.

I glared at him.

'You have just purchased a few new pants of size 38. What will happen to them? I would suggest you to get them altered to 36 and wear them for some time. You can buy new ones when your size is permanent and stable.'

She was making sense, but I was disappointed as this was my first reward of sweating it out at the gym. I felt let down and she sensed the mood.

'Go ahead and buy this.'

'But then I will also get then new ones altered,' she added quickly.

I have learnt to take one battle at a time in my career. So, I did not argue on the altered trousers and was happy with a small victory of buying a new one.

One question that has always bugged me is whether to buy a pleated or a flat front trouser. Initially, my trainer had told me that the upper abs is easier to reduce than the lower ones. But over the months, I have begun to realize the reverse. My trainer could not believe that this could also be true. I have proven to be a unique case in his career. Not only this, his prediction about biceps has also proved to be wrong in my case, as my triceps have taken shape much before the biceps were formed. He considered it as a new learning.

As my lower abdomen has begun to look flatter, the flat front trousers were the logical choice. But when I tried some of these, my stubborn upper abdomen looked quite bloated under my shirt. In pleated pants, my lower abs and legs appeared more baggy and loose. After trying a few brands of trousers, I could find a near perfect flat front pair of pants, which did not bulge over the belt.

> **Tip!** During the journey of fitness, different body parts take different amounts of time to shape up. So, be patient and try various brands before choosing a right outfit which can do proper justice to your transforming body.

As time progressed and I settled well with size 36, the time had come for me to find a way to explore more brands of trousers. I deviously devised excuses concerning the altered ones alleging that only the waist was altered and not the whole leg, or the leg was not tapered enough and so on. She insisted on going slow as it had just been a month or so. By the end of it, she was fed up and gave up, and soon I had my new wardrobe much to my wife's dismay.

I continued my fitness regime with a new excitement. A good number of months passed by but the probable issues which my wife had voiced became apparent. I could make out that my belt required a new intermediate hole. The current belt was promptly replaced with a new one. This could have been happy news, but in my case, I knew what it meant. Size 36 also began to loosen around my waist. This meant that my wife was right to advise me to be patient in this fitness journey and continue with altered pants for some more time. Now, I was in a dilemma.

'How do I break this good news?' I wondered.

'What is the proof that I will need a size 34 instead now?'

On my next visit to the mall, I secretly tried size 34 which fitted me well. I thought for a moment on how to face my wife and decided to follow the principle—aggression is the best defence.

'Look my hard work has started to pay faster. I reduced my waist size again. Size 34 fitted perfectly.' I looked at her confidently.

To my surprise she was very happy and said, 'I could see your dedication and this is the positive outcome.'

But I wondered how could she let go off the opportunity to not remind me about her earlier suggestion.

'This time I will get your new 36 ones altered to 34,' she added.

I did not insist on new pants and wanted to wait for some more time.

> **Caution** The loss in weight is not uniform but happens in cycles of plateau and weight-loss. Before you change your wardrobe, make sure that you have entered the period of plateau where your weight has stabilized for some time as the new normal.

By now, my upper body had also begun to change and

my shirt size had come down from 42 to 40. Casual fit to regular fit was an obvious transition, but then something else happened to my wardrobe. I always wore bold colours and designs till the time I chose my own clothes. I had gradually begun to depend on my wife's choices as the shirts that she chose were appreciated at work. I remember my first birthday after marriage when she had gifted me an office shirt and a tie, and I just did not like the shirt. Since then she had stopped giving me surprise gifts. When she found that I had started liking her choice of clothes, she got me two shirts as a surprise on my recent birthday. This was the second time she has given me a surprise gift since our marriage. She had told me that one was of her liking and the other was what I usually wear. She advised me to wear the shirt of her liking to work the next day. To my surprise, I was appreciated for the shirt and I shared it with my wife. She was certainly happy. After a few days, I wore the one of my choice, and there were no comments.

My wardrobe had begun to have more clothes with hues of blues, blacks, greys and whites. It was difficult for me to accept this transformation, as for me bright colours represent happiness and positivity. Then, I changed.

> **Tip!** One wears any garment for two reasons—for comfort and to enhance their appearance. Your choice of outfit should accommodate both.

Once my wife commented, 'You should see the huge pile of old clothes that I have taken out to donate to charity and then decide to go shopping in future.'

I simply mumbled 'okay', but did not tell her that I had been trying out slim fit shirts hoping to fit into a one soon and the donation pile will grow bigger.

Around this time, I had begun to get an urge to become stylish and trendy. Anything looks good on you when you are getting into shape, so it is natural to try the trendy stuff and align with the latest fashion. Instead of rummaging for shirts that would conceal my fat, I could now hunt for those which could enhance my physique. The only challenge for me was to buy stuff which was appropriate for my age and not simply because it was in vogue. Though over the years the rules of dressing for different age groups have relaxed, still there are things that look good only on youngsters.

Soon the time came when not only my waist size reduced to 32 but the size of my shirts also came down to 38. Some people do not reduce their shirt size to appear broad and strong. Initially, I too hesitated to buy slim fit shirts as they could make me look boyish, but then regular fits were too loose for me. I convinced myself that it would be an injustice towards the hard-earned physique if it were not clad in well-fitted clothes.

Around that time, I had started to like one of the European menswear brand of clothes as they fitted me better, giving a contemporary look. I had met them and agreed to do a brand influencer video. They were supposed to ask me some questions about my professional journey clubbed with a few shoots of their store as well as trying out a few shirts. Of course, I had to tell them about what I liked with the brand. The video came out quite well and it got around 15,000 views. This certainly was a pleasant unexpected milestone in my journey of fitness.

As mentioned earlier, grooming is certainly important for your career. Even though, your office is not a place to flaunt your clothes, but proper, clean and well-fitted ones enhance the personality. When you are fit and wear clothes as per the occasion, you are setting your own style statement.

> **Tip!** Spending money in keeping abreast with the latest trend is certainly important for certain professions, but for many others it is good to follow the latest trend without splurging money. In addition, by being fit, you can carry off anything suitable, so it need not be expensive.

Skin: My employees started seeing me as a person who is trying to reverse the ageing process. I was secretly happy on hearing this. When I began my fitness, I just wanted to lose a few kilograms of weight. But over the years, rather than being complacent with what is being achieved slowly and steadily, the body itself started taking me towards the so called 'reverse ageing'. How you dress yourself and present yourself is very important, but your skin plays a major role in reverse ageing. I am not an expert on how to keep a good skin, but here are some of my experiences.

Six pack abs has entered everyone's vocabulary and a dream for anyone who joins a gym. I too was curious to know the secret of achieving it, even though moderately cognizant that it was not my cup of tea. I asked my trainer, 'Attaining six pack abs will be quite difficult, but do people get four pack abs?'

'Yes sir, there are people in our gym who have four pack abs,' he replied.

'Oh! So that is possible,' I said.

'Yes, but are you asking about yourself?' he enquired.

My trainer was looking at me as if I am an exotic animal in a zoo.

'You focus on general fitness rather than on how many

pack of abs you would have,' he continued.

He tried to brush away my question.

'It will be a long journey, currently your body fat is around 30 per cent. When it goes lower than 20 per cent, you will begin to see the abs. As the body fat continues to reduce, you will be able to see two packs, and then four pack abs. But why do you ask, sir? Why do you need it?' he asked.

'I don't need it, but I should be equipped with such information,' I replied.

'Sir, it will not be visible even if you get it,' he laughed. I felt insulted and did not join his laughter.

He quickly became serious and added, 'When your waist starts to reduce, the loose skin due to your age will take quite a while to shrink and probably might not shrink to the extent to show your abs.'

He was right. Even after years, and I have journeyed far enough, a clear view of the taut abs is still hidden under loose skin, which is tightening slowly.

> **Caution** Cardiovascular exercises help in burning the calories and reduce the weight, but if not done together with some weight lifting exercises, it will leave the skin loose.

I was not concerned about the loose skin at the waist, but I had seen people who have undergone weight loss with loose skin and wrinkles or stretch marks on their faces and around their necks. This was a cause of worry for me. Fat from the face is the last one to go, and therefore, a chiseled face without loose skin is a visible symbol of fitness.

When I had started to lose fat around my neck, much before the fat I lost from my face, wrinkles had begun to appear around the neck. I was very worried about that. I always took inputs from multiple people on various things and based on such inputs, around that time, I was advised to start pull-up and chin-up. These were very difficult exercises. It took me a few months to start doing a few counts in the proper form. I could see that the skin around my neck had started to look tighter, and most importantly, the fat from the face had begun to reduce fast too, without leaving any wrinkles or folds in the skin. Pull-ups and chin-ups helped in toning my neck and face.

The best nutrient for the skin is sweat. The article 'Live Long and Perspire', published in tothegloss.com, provides a list of benefits of sweating. It says that sweating not only helps in the removal of impurities from your skin, but it also protects it from bacteria such as E. coli and Staphylococcus aureus by secreting a rather nifty natural antibiotic called Dermcidin. It mentions further that it is good for the whole skin, and therefore steam rooms and sauna helps in sweating to make the skin look better.

I tried not to wipe the sweat unless it was necessary. Let the sweat get absorbed by your skin. It is better to pat the sweat rather than wipe it off. Sweat seemed to make my hair look better which I noticed later. The reason is that it unclogs the hair follicles, allowing the new hair to grow. I do not take a shower immediately after the gym, but wear a warm jacket that makes me sweat some more and then take a shower after about 30 minutes of completing the exercise.

Tip! Sweat is not only good for your skin but also for your hair. Try not to wipe off immediately, but let it stay on the skin. Wash it off after some time to avoid any skin disease.

Sweat is the best natural moisturizer for the skin, but the body needs a thorough cleansing to prevent any body odour and skin disease. However, you cannot depend upon sweat all the time for your skin to be moisturized. Skin needs constant care. Using a moisturizer separately or together with some sun protection cream is good for the skin. If exercising outdoors, a sun protection cream should be applied in a way so that it does not run into your eyes. It also helps if you could wash your face a couple of times with plain water. But then these are external tips. You should also drink sufficient water and eat plenty of fruits and salads to keep the skin fresh. Don't forget to get a good sleep and adequate rest.

Have you wondered if smoking affects your skin? Smoking clearly helps in reducing weight as nicotine suppresses the appetite, but that should not be the reason for this habit. The side effect of smoking is not only restricted to faster ageing or the cause for cancer, because of which the pack carries the warning 'Smoking is injurious to health'. It is also because 'smoking cigarettes destroys collagen and elastin and decreases levels of estrogen, which is necessary to keep skin firm,' says New York City dermatologist Fredric Brandt. Smoking causes the skin to lose its firmness, which makes you look older than you actually are.

> **Caution** Smoking reduces the elasticity of your skin, while alcohol along with high intake of refined sugar and salt causes water retention leading to puffiness of face.

How does exercise help in the quality of your skin?

'We tend to focus on the cardiovascular benefits of physical activity, and those are important. But anything that promotes healthy circulation also helps keep your skin healthy and vibrant,' says dermatologist Ellen Marmur, in Peter Jaret's article 'Exercise for Healthy Skin' in www.webmd.com.

In the article, says Marmur, 'If you have dermatological conditions such as acne, rosacea, or psoriasis, you may need to take special care to keep your skin protected while exercising. But don't let skin problems prevent you from being active. Blood carries oxygen and nutrients to working cells throughout the body, including the skin.' In addition to providing oxygen, blood flow also helps carry away waste products, including free radicals, from working cells. Contrary to some claims, exercise doesn't detoxify the skin. The job of neutralizing toxins belongs mostly to the liver. 'But by increasing blood flow, a bout of exercise helps flush cellular debris out of the system,' Marmur tells WebMD. 'You can think of it as cleansing your skin from the inside.' The article recommended to avoid doing exercise during the hottest time of the day to avoid sun exposure or sun burn which can increase the risk of skin cancer and aid in rapid ageing.

Here, it is important to share the importance of a massage. Much before I joined the gym I used to get an ayurvedic massage once or twice a month. My masseur has been coming to my home for more than a decade now. When I joined the gym, they insisted on the importance of massage as it relaxes the muscles from soreness. Some gyms do offer spas as well. A massage not only helps in relaxing muscles, but it also nourishes the skin. Skin dryness, which is common during winter, might need an increased frequency of massage. My masseur complemented me whenever I lost more weight or my muscles seemed to have toned up further.

He told me long back that I looked fine and did not need a fitness regime further, but I continued. When he hiked his charges, I told him that he should be rather offering a discount as my body surface area has reduced significantly now.

> **Tip!** Getting a massage is an added benefit to relax the muscle and reduce soreness caused due to exercising.

I was under the impression that the fat on the face is responsible for glow and shine. Exercises will reduce the fat percentage and with the increase of lean mass, the face might lose the sheen. I was also worried about the loose facial skin giving way to wrinkles, adding years to my face. The trainer assured me that balanced exercise will not lead to such things. I took up the challenge of going ahead to further reduce my body fat. As I started to progress, I noticed some uniformity in the texture of my face and was somewhat ashamed to ask anyone except my wife and she said, 'I can't make out as I see you daily, but whatever it is, it certainly is not going in a wrong direction.'

As time passed, I was more convinced of the changes on my face and curiously searched the web about it. I found an article 'How Diet and Exercise can Improve your Complexion' published in *The Telegraph*. In this article, Katy Young quoted Dalton Wong, a celebrity trainer, saying,

> The correct exercises will help you tone your skin in much the same way you tone your muscles. The key in training to tone your skin is to focus on increasing lean muscle mass. As we age, our skin naturally loses its plump, youthful layer of fat. But if you exercise the

right way, you can build up muscle which gives that same volatizing effect. It's the lean muscle mass that sits just under the surface which can create a lifted, taut looking, skin.

Bang on, this is what I was experiencing. And then one day, one fitness enthusiast in my office was talking to me about some work-related challenge and towards the end the topic moved to fitness.

In our official mailing system, every employee ID is tied to their name and photo. My picture was some seven to eight years old. He commented, 'You must be very regular and methodical in doing your exercise, else it is difficult to get such a uniformity on the face not only at your age, but for younger folks too.'

I smiled as I didn't know how to respond at that moment.

He quickly added, 'Why don't you replace your old picture with your current one?'

'I will not. It reminds me how far I have come in the journey of fitness and feel happy about it. This picture encourages me not to go back as well.'

First, he smiled and then looked at me seriously and with a deep sigh he said, 'But you should understand the problem with the new employees. One day when you passed by the cafeteria, a new employee in my team asked which team did you belong to. Everyone around him started laughing, and once he came to know you, he said that your picture does not match you at all.'

He began to laugh.

'If I decide to change I will change, but I don't plan to do so at present.'

Such conversations reminded me of the same article

which also said, 'to improve your skin, you'll want to focus on resistance training, where you're using your own bodyweight to challenge your muscles. Lunges, pushups, and planking are examples of resistance exercises.'

Some consider sculpted face is the most visible reflection of your fitness. I have come across many who are regular in their exercise regime, but they still do not have a sculpted face. The new trend is to have a slim face, but then it also depends on the individual to decide to go for it or not. I once met a person who had maintained himself and wanted to get fitter but was adamant to not let fitness impact his face. His reason was that, 'My girlfriend likes my face a lot and she told me not to do more exercise as it will impact my face.'

I was somewhat puzzled. Cautiously I said, 'Sure, the beauty lies in the eye of the beholder, but in my opinion, with a slight weight gain your face will become plump and you will look more aged than what you are.'

He looked at me puzzled and did not reply. After a few months he saw me and came running to me. He asked, 'Tell me how to reduce the fat. I want to shed a few kgs, and I know my face has bloated too.'

'Why, doesn't your girlfriend like you anymore?' I teased him.

'She is plump, so she does not mind it at all,' he smiled and then quickly added, 'But I am not able to see myself in the mirror. I have to reduce weight but most importantly a lot from face.'

By now, many things started to happen to me. There were small but noticeable things that are sometimes difficult to explain. During my search to find answers to some of these things, I came across another article, which matched some of my observations. Written by Catherine Guthrie on expereincelife.com, titled '8 Ways Exercise Makes Your Skin Gorgeous' and published in April 2010, it said,

> The rewards of exercise extend far beyond slimming down or adding muscle tone. Dozens of subtle changes visibly revamp the body and the psyche in ways scientists are only beginning to understand. Maybe your skin looks brighter, your step is springier or you're more confident at work. Such small victories may go unnoticed by unobservant exercisers, but those on the lookout for these benefits will find them every bit as valid as gains measured by scales and calipers.

You might be wondering whether these are applicable to male, female or to both. First, let us try to understand the difference between male and female skin. Rita Lee is the founder and author of a skin care blog. Such differences were detailed in the April 2014 issue of www.justaboutskin.com. She wrote,

> Male skin is actually the same as female skin until puberty. There's really no difference in children. After puberty, male and female skin starts to diverge due to sex hormones. The skin differences are both structural and chemical. Not only a man's skin is about 20 per cent thicker than that of a woman's, it has more collagen, and therefore, ages slowly. Men also age slower because they have more facial hair. More hair follicles mean less crepey wrinkling on the cheeks.

The article continued to state,

> The skin's elasticity is the same for men and women. Men produce more oil. Oil lubricates and moisturizes skin, which is why men are typically less prone to dry skin. Men also sweat more than women, and therefore more bacteria, which leads to more odour. Men lose water faster than women. This is water loss due to the natural evaporation of water from skin, not sweating. Greater water loss makes re-hydration important for men.

The article further writes that women have lighter, cooler skin than men and have more fat, and any skin injury heals faster in women than in men.

The above differences are factually correct, but it did not mention that exercise will work one way for male skin and another for female skin. So, with proper exercise, having the right food and keeping well hydrated helps to improve facial skin for both men and women.

> **Tip!** Clean eating like enough salad and fresh fruit, taking plenty of water and having a good fitness regime triggers a good amount of sweat. A good sleep also makes your face glow.

Neither has anyone suggested any facial exercises to me at the gym, nor have I asked for them. There are exercises to get a sculpted face. It is also true that everyone does not want to have a sculpted face, because of the age-old belief that sculpted face appears weak therefore giving an unhealthy look. Also for some, sculpted face means having deep lines and appearing older than they actually are.

Sculpted face was neither my agenda nor a desire, as my goal was to reduce the weight. The sculpted look began to show on my face too due to that balance in my workout routine done in the right way. There are many facial exercises. Some of them are mentioned in 'Cheek Exercises for a Sculpted face' by Sarabethasaff, written on blog.udemy.com in May 2014, like X and O, Cheek Lift, Fish Lips, Puffy Cheeks, etc. But then, the article also said, 'Believe it or not, smiling widely and holding it for 10 seconds at a time can be a great way to work your cheek muscles. Best of all, you never have to feel foolish while you perform this exercise, and it's guaranteed to help lift your mood as well.'

I did not try any of these, but I do one exercise my mother taught me a good number of years back. The exercise is to inhale through the mouth and hold it by stretching the cheeks like a balloon. I continued to do it a couple of times per day and it helped. It is said that the face is the mirror of your health.

> **Tip!** Face reflects your health. Balancing cardiovascular and strength exercises will help in reduction of fat from the face that happens towards the end of a fitness journey.

There was a new member at the gym and seemed to be in a better shape. He also had some knowledge about fitness.

He had taken control of one of the gym equipment and was not happy using it. He looked around and saw me and asked, 'Bro, can you help me? I can't see any trainers around.'

'Sure. You are young and you could do it this way. I do it somewhat easily,' I explained to him how it could be done both ways.

He looked puzzled and asked me, 'Why do you mention

age? You must be just a couple of years older than me,' he said. The person seemed to be in early 30s.

'You must be 35 or a little older,' he continued.

I smiled and did not say anything. I went back to do my own exercise.

We would bump into each other few days in a week and exchange pleasantries. Slowly, we started to have some more interactions. He continued to address me as 'Bro'.

One day, another trainer came to me, while I was talking to him, and asked,

'Sir, my trainee wants to talk to you about a few floor exercises that you just did. She is wondering if she could take a few tips from you about these floor exercises.' He pointed at the person he was talking about. She was a regular to gym for a good number of months.

'I have not advised anyone, and I might not be the right one for youngsters. Why can't you advise her?' I replied.

'Sir, she said that the exercises are not helping her much, but they are helping you. So, she wants to take a few inputs. But, I told her that you are quite senior and might not be willing to guide you... Let it be, sir. I will help her. I just wanted to let her know that I did ask you.'

The trainer walked away and left me in a dilemma—to help or not. The guy who was listening to the conversation interrupted my thoughts.

'May I know your name?' he asked.

I told him my name and went to that trainer, from whom by now I took only occasional inputs, and asked him to go and help that girl.

As I came back to my exercise, the guy, whom I was talking to, came running.

'Sir, I kept addressing you as "Bro" all the time. But

then, you don't look like a sir to me.'

By then, he had looked me up on the Internet.

We laughed and talked more and he continued to call me 'Bro'.

Hygiene: Grooming does not mean just a change in the wardrobe, but also keeping a good hygiene. Hygiene does not only mean washing one's hands regularly or using a sanitizer periodically, but taking care of oneself and one's surroundings for a healthy living. Regular exercise will certainly enhance the hygiene. For maintaining hygiene, body odour, clean clothes and good upkeep of facial hair for men are some of the other things which should be taken care of. As far as the surroundings are considered, we must keep fitness facilities also neat and clean. I have seen a few posters inside some gyms which said, 'Don't smell like fish', 'Mind your neighbhours', 'Keep the gym equipment clean', etc. Some organizations have in-house facilities and people tend to use it during working hours. Whether you have a gym at office or you don't, maintaining good hygiene at workplace is equally important.

> **Tip!** At workplace, we do not work alone but in a team, and it is important that one should not repulse another by poor hygiene.

In my first job, I was assigned a project under the guidance of a senior. We had a few more team members and they had been with the company for a few years. My guide was quite senior in the organization, so it was a privilege to work with him and I was quite excited. He had a fixed daily routine; for the first few hours, he would do his own work like attending meetings and then from late morning till early afternoon, he would review our work and again attend some more meetings. His review in the middle of the day served two purposes: First, it made us work hard from the morning itself as a review was awaited, and second, any changes which he would suggest had to be taken care of in the same evening. So practically, this meant that most of the days, I had to work longer hours. That was still OK. The problem was that my review was scheduled immediately after his lunch break. He had raw onions with his lunch, which made the meeting a torturous time for me, without any escape. A ray of hope appeared after a few months when one of my colleagues went on leave. I took that slot and soon made it a permanent swap before he could return, saving me from the bad odour. As a new trend, workplaces have started few fitness activities. Therefore, the habit of not taking care of the bad odour affects others participating in the fitness activities, making it unbearable for them.

Though the awareness to maintain hygiene at the workplace is increasing, but still more has to be done. For example, there are people who don't change their shirts for two days, even in a hot and humid weather. You should use deodorants or perfumes and wear clean shirts. The challenge during the winter season is different. It is assumed that as the amount of sweat generated is very little, so one shirt could be worn for many days. It is advisable to judge for yourself and when in doubt don't repeat the shirt. In winters, people forget that winter garments also need to be cleaned occasionally, if not frequently. Most of the time, jackets and hoodies which are used frequently must be cleaned too. This is also true for any merchandise which is provided by the organization to the employees. Most of the times just because the company has provided shirts or hoodies does not mean that you can wear them every day without a wash. If you are using the office gym or cycling or jogging to it, make sure you shower and change your attire to maintain proper hygiene at workplace.

> **Caution** Be aware that any bad odour could spread faster in an air-conditioned office due to air circulation and might impact working together as a team.

Height: Does exercise increase one's height? In teens, stretch exercises can help grow the height, but there is also hearsay that heavy weight lifting by teens might stunt their heights. No study has ever proved this assumption, but if not done under proper supervision, it may pose as a problem. Coming to adults, it is also seen that exercise may help one to grow, mostly for those who are in their 20s. Height is determined by genes, nutrition, limb bones and spinal conditions. A question came to my mind that if at any age one can grow or shrink our individual body parts like biceps, triceps, etc., through exercises, why can't we do the same for the full body. I tried to find out the answer, but could not. Certainly, exercise improves overall health of the body, but it does not help in improving the height, because the body is made of many muscles and it is impossible to target all at the same time with the same intensity.

But why do some people look taller than they are while others look shorter than they actually are?

It is your body proportion that matters. Hardly anyone has an ideal body proportion. We make it worse by letting the unwanted fat get deposited at the wrong places that makes our body look more disproportionate. Lack of exercise keeps making things worse, and the problem gets further compounded by sedentary jobs which result in bad postures. Walking straight for many becomes a challenge. All these combined will make the person's height appear to be quite less than it actually is.

> **Tip!** For those who spend the majority of their time inside the office must focus on ergonomics, which is very important for a right posture and take a small walk periodically rather than sitting for a long time in the cubicle.

I could see myself how my overall body proportion and perceived heights went down with the reduction in fitness level as I aged from 20s to 30s to 40s. Exercising really helped me in reducing the excess fat from various body parts and giving a slimmer and more proportionate look. This, together with walking straight, helped in building a perception of being taller than I am.

Bollywood stars have taken up fitness 1990s onwards. Have you noticed the physique of the stars in the 1990s? They might seem fitter and taller to you nowadays.

In the article '8 Exercises Which Can Make You Gorgeous', published in April 2010 on www.experiencelife.com, Catherine Guthrie has also spoken about the benefits of exercise to increase stature. She has given an example of Annie Appleby, 45, a yoga instructor and founder of YogaForce LLC in San Francisco, who had taken up yoga as a means to relieve stress. After a few years of practice, she went for a check-up which showed effects of yoga. When the doctor measured her height, it was found that she'd grown an inch and a half. 'No one has studied precisely why exercise makes you look taller, but activities that stretch and strengthen muscles at the same time, like yoga or Pilates, can correct bad posture and therefore increase height,' says Dan Bradley, MD, an orthopedic surgeon at the Texas Back Institute in Denton. Hunching makes a group of muscles contract and others lengthen, he explains, which decreases the height. 'If you actively work to bring muscles back into balance, your back will lengthen, your posture will improve and you can grow taller.'

Yes, exercise does help you to appear taller than you are by correcting the posture and shaping up the body.

However, this change in my physique also came with a few side effects. I was being noticed now—at malls, theatres, cinema halls and other public places—which was an anomaly for me. It took me some time to get used to this new reality. Occasionally, it was quite amusing though. I teased my wife, 'For decades, people have noticed you and now it's my turn.'

She smiled and said, 'All your hard work is paying off and you deserve such attention.'

All the above measures like focusing on style, taking care of my skin, maintaining a good hygiene and right posture has enhanced how I look and it would definitely enhance yours too.

Let me tell you about an episode of my childhood. I am the youngest among three siblings. On seeing my transformation, my sister told me about an incident that took place many years ago.

I was around two years old and my sister was going to a party with her friends in the neighbourhood. It was evening and my mother asked my sister to take me along.

'Him? No Ma, I cannot take him to the party,' my sister protested.

'Why not? Not that he will disturb you,' my mother told her.

'No, Ma,' she was adamant.

My mother was astonished and asked her, 'Why are you not listening? Do I ask you to take him out every day? I have some work today and the nanny has also left for the day. It will be of great help to me if you take your brother along,' she explained.

She pointed to my elder brother and offered to take him instead. But not me as according to her, I was quite 'ugly'.

I was quite amused when I heard her narrate the story, but she continued.

'Here you are an epitome of ugly duckling story,' she laughed and complemented me, as now the tides have turned and both my older siblings are fighting the battle of the bulge.

It has been a long journey from being an ugly duckling to what I am now. The only regret is that I could have taken up fitness a couple of decades earlier. But at this stage of my life, it certainly is a big satisfaction and achievement. My sincere advice would be to not wait that long to undertake the journey of fitness, as the younger you are the easier it is to transform yourself into a better you.

SPECIAL SECTION #4

Maintaining Fitness at Home and while on Travel

Vinod Channa
Celebrity fitness trainer (certified) and winner of multiple awards

After a thorough study of the lifestyle of different people and continuous training for years, I have realized that there are many things that people do not understand or aren't aware of when it comes to the term 'fitness'. They seem to indulge in exercises when they face physical problems due to the lack of movement. This is when they rush to the gyms or take up other fitness classes. Once they join, they are appointed a trainer who based on his or her learning and experience, rather than having an idea about the person's lifestyle, instructs the trainee.

Trainer Issue

Most of the trainers fail to consider or foresee probable medical problems or issues that may arise while training. This is because most of the current trainers impose whatever training they have learned from their academy, but do not engage in preparing a routine based on the client's lifestyle or requirement.

Lifestyle Issue

Another issue is that people do not have time to go to the gym due to the competitive nature of the corporate industry. This lifestyle also makes them tired and fatigued due to incorrect eating habits and sitting continuously for long hours. In this way, they not only lose strength, stamina and flexibility, but it also affects their speed, mobility, agility, endurance, power, impact bearing capacity and mind and body coordination. All these can be achieved from different fitness techniques like strength with weight training, flexibility with dynamic and static stretches and yoga, speed and agility from functional training, parkour, gymnastic, callisthenics and other such training. There are other conditioning and balancing techniques achieved from gadget training like TRX, Bosuball, Swiss Ball, Kettle bell, etc. Let me explain some of the exercises which can be easily done at home.

Body weight exercises that can be done at home as per your body parts:

Chest

1. Knee push-up (half push-up)
2. Full push-up
3. Spider push-up
4. Cross fly push-up
5. Single hand push-up
6. Shoulder tap push-up
7. Clap push-up

Back

1. Superman
2. Cross superman
3. Lying alternate leg raise and both leg raise
4. Cat Camel pose

Shoulder

1. Pyramid push-up
2. Pyramid push-up shoulder tap
3. Pyramid side walk
4. Quadrupedal walk

Triceps

1. Triceps dips
2. Crab walk
3. Close grip tricep push-up

Legs

1. Free Squat
2. Squat and jump
3. Squat hold
4. Squat pulse
5. Lunges
6. Jumping lunges
7. Cross lunges
8. Forward and back lunges
9. Lying down leg curl
10. Hip thruster
11. Calf both leg and single leg

Abs

1. Crunches
2. Leg raises
3. Toe touch crunches
4. Cross crunches
5. Plank
6. Side plank

7. Elbow palm plank
8. Mountain climber

Total body workout (dynamic exercises)

1. Burpees
2. Burpees with push-up
3. Single hand and single leg burpees
4. Jumping Jacks
5. Knee tuck jump

If you have only 30 minutes with you to spare, you can mix and match all body part exercises, especially those for bigger muscles like legs, back and chest, and if you are looking for more fat loss, then make a schedule as follows:

Day 1

1. Free squat
2. Squat and jump
3. Knee bend push-up or full push-up
4. Tiger walk
5. Toe touch abdominal plank hold 30 seconds
6. Triceps dips

*Perform all 10-20 counts three times.

Day 2

Cardio: walking, jogging, dancing, aerobics, cycling, etc. 30 minutes to more than an hour depending on the fat percentage and the level of fitness.

Day 3

- Tiger walk
- Squat and jump
- Spider push up

- Jumping lung
- 90 Degree crunches
- Mountain climber
- Plank Elbow palm

Perform all 10-20 count 3 times

Day 4

Cardio (walking/jogging/dancing/aerobics/cycling, etc.) 30 minutes to more than an hour depending on the fat percentage and fitness.

Day 5

- Jumping Jack
- Knee tuck jump and burpees
- Superman pose turn and toe touch
- Plank Hold (30 seconds to 1 minutes) with 3 way mountain climber
- Quadrupedal walk

Perform all 10-20 count 3 times

If you are really short of time and you have only 15 minutes to workout. Try the following exercises:

Tabata

Tabata training was discovered by Japanese scientist Dr Izumi Tabata and a team of researchers from the National Institute of Fitness and Sports in Tokyo. Tabata and his team in their research concluded that high-intensity interval training has more impact on both the aerobic and anaerobic systems. Short intervals between exercises utilize maximum oxygen and give you a good intensity workout at home. This is a more cardio-based workout.

Tabata training

Each exercise in each Tabata workout lasts only four minutes, but it's likely to be one of the longest four minutes you've ever endured. The structure of the programme is as follows:

> Workout hard for 20 seconds
> Rest for 10 seconds
> Complete 8 rounds

You push yourself as hard as you can for 20 seconds and rest for 10 seconds. This is one set. Likewise, complete 8 sets of each exercise in 4 minutes. Take a one-minute rest after completing 6 sets.

You can do pretty much any exercise you wish. You can do squats, push-ups, burpees or any other exercise that works your large muscle groups like legs, back or chest. Tabata generally has a 2:1 ratio.

Example of Tabata workout 1:

- Push-ups
- Free squats
- Mountain climbers

Start with push-ups. Perform them for 20 seconds. Rest for 10 seconds, and then again do push-ups for 20 seconds and rest 10 seconds. In this way continue for 4 minutes. Then, rest for 1 minute after the completion of 8 sets.

Next, move on to squats and repeat the sequence of 20 seconds on, 10 seconds off. Once you finish 8 sets of squats, rest for 1 minute, and then do mountain climbers.

This completes your 12-minute workout schedule.

Tabata is a great way to get a quick workout if you're short of time, you need to switch routine or you want to improve endurance and speed. Incorporate this type of workout into your fitness routine and see the results. Also, note that selection of workout is very important and quite challenging if you have a desired target to achieve.

You can also make variations in the same ratio of 2:1 by changing exercises in each set—doing push-ups for 20 seconds, resting for 10 seconds, moving on to squats for 20 seconds, again resting for 10 seconds. Again, switch back to push-ups for 20 seconds with 10 seconds of rest and move on to squats till you complete 4 minutes. After completion of 4 minutes, rest for 1 minute and take up different exercises.

Following exercises can be performed to cover the whole body:

For lower body:

- Squats
- Lunges
- Leg Kicking

For Upper Body:

- Push-ups
- Variation of push-ups
- Superman pose
- Hip raises

For abs:

- Crunches
- Plank

For complete body movements:

- Burpees
- Side to side jump
- Knee tuck jump

HIIT for 20 to 40 Minutes Workout

HIIT is High Intensity Interval Training, where the scheduling generally requires you to workout for 30 seconds to 2 minutes, followed by a 30-second to 2-minute recovery period (depending on the work duration).

HIIT is more often in a ratio of 1:1 or 1:2. This means 1 minute of workout, one minute of rest, or 1 minute of workout and 2 minutes of rest.

You can mix it up and do 2:1, meaning 2 minutes of workout and 1 minute of rest.

Generally, harder the workout, longer the rest will have to be.

HIIT workouts can be anywhere from 20–40 minutes.

The following workout can be performed:

When performed vigorously and with variety, callisthenics can provide the benefits of muscular and aerobic conditioning, in addition to improving skills such as balance, agility and coordination.

Other than the above mentioned exercises, the following can also be performed:

1. Push-up
2. Squat
3. Crunches
4. Plank hold

10 repetitions; 3 sets

1. Squat and jump
2. Spider push-up
3. Mountain climb

You can mix and match in this way, with minimum of 20 repetitions.

If you have a treadmill at home and you can buy a few dumbbells, say 5 kg, 7.5 kg and 10 kg, you can also do some exercises at home.

If you have treadmill at home you can jog on alternate days or whenever you are talking on the cell phone, you can walk and talk instead of sitting at one place. Also, 15 to 20 minutes of jogging post-workout speeds up the process of fat-loss.

If you can buy dumbells as per the fitness level, and you can perform following workouts:

- Shoulder overhead press

- Front and side lateral raises
- Chest press
- Dumbbell fly
- Single hand dumbbell row
- Bend over dumbbell row
- Biceps curl
- Triceps curl
- Squats
- Lunges
- Step up
- Crunches with dumbells

The eating pattern depends upon what you eat before the exercise:

If you eat more than 2 hours before workout, you are allowed to eat protein, carbohydrate and essential fat together.

If you eat one hour before the workout, you are allowed to eat carbohydrate and protein.

If you are eating 20-30 minutes before workout, you are allowed to eat simple carbohydrates like fruits and sweet potatoes.

In a post-workout meal, you must eat protein and carbohydrate together within 20 minutes of the workout.

Carbohydrates again recover your energy and protein helps to build your muscles, which breaks down during the workout.

Breathing Pattern

A) The following breathing pattern should followed for weight training.
1. Always inhale before starting a particular exercise.
2. Always exhale against gravity and against resistance.
B) Yoga and Pilates have different breathing patterns as per the movements.

Note: If you do not understand breathing patterns, instead of performing the wrong pattern of breathing, breathe normally throughout the exercise.

Travellers' Workout

Generally, when you are travelling for long hours or frequently via airway, train, bus or any other mode of transport, you sit for long hours and sleep in an uncomfortable positions. These lead to stiffness in the knee, back and neck. Travellers usually complain of some discomfort in these body parts during and after their journey.

If you are travelling frequently or for long hours, you must do regular exercises to improve strength, mobility and flexibility for muscles and joints not used while travelling. If you do not take proper care of these body parts, they will lose strength, mobility and flexibility, and you will find it difficult to cope with day-to-day activities. Due to the stiffness, there are high chances of the muscle to wear and tear and the joints to dislocate. You might not be able to perform as per your potential and there will always be some kind of pain, pull or other such hindrances.

To get back what you have lost and to prevent such happening, following are few easy exercises that can be performed while you are travelling:

Start with the following joint mobility moves:

1. Waist rotation
2. Shoulder rotation
3. Ankle rotation
4. Wrist rotation
5. Torso bends
6. Back stretch
7. Side to side bends

Then, do the following exercises:

1. Cat camel pose
2. Glute kickback
3. Quadrupedal walk–5 steps forwards and 5 backwards, start with 4 to 5 round.

4. Free squats 90 degree 10 reps
5. Rock bottom squats 10 reps
6. Squat hold 10 to 30 seconds and squat side walk
7. Half push-up or full push-up 10 repetitions with mountain climber
8. Superman pose 10 reps, 10 seconds hold 3 times
9. Hip raise 10 reps 10 seconds hold
10. Sitting lunges
11. Plank hold 10 to 30 seconds
12. Toe touch with immediate superman
13. Side leg kicking and back leg kicking

You can pick any 5 exercises from the list and divide it over 3-4 days a week.

Then, do the following post-workout stretches:

- Hamstring stretches
- Glute stretches
- Back stretches

SEVEN

Sexual, Physical and Mental Benefits

Many a times, I have been asked about the relation between fitness and sex life. Initially, I ignored this question but later I too became curious. I could not ask such questions to my trainer, so my knowledge on this subject is mostly based on the content available on the Internet. Let us first understand our sex hormones before we can delve further into the topic.

Male Sex Hormone

Testosterone is a male hormone produced primarily by the testicles. It does play a large role in male sexuality and reproduction. It not only affects factors like sexual and reproductive functioning, muscle mass, hair growth, but also maintains bone density, levels of red blood cells and a sense of well-being.

Does testosterone reduce with age?

Yes, many studies have found that from 30s, a man's testosterone level begins to decline. When testosterone is reducing in men, the female hormone estrogen starts to increase. Obesity is also a cause for reduction of testosterone as written by Scott Issacs, in his book *Hormonal Balance:*

How to Lose Weight By Understanding Your Hormones and Metabolism. Issacs says,

> Testosterone levels vary throughout the day. Levels are typically highest in the morning and lowest in the afternoon. Research has found that strength-training workouts may have a bigger effect on testosterone in the evening. As a result, the brief boost from your exercise session might be even bigger if you schedule it after work instead of early in the morning.

Tip! Age and obesity cause reduction in testosterone. Exercise will boost testosterone and thereby improve overall health including sexual life.

I do my exercise after work, not because I knew the above study earlier but because I am a morning person and I spend my most productive morning time at work. I do agree with the above study but only when I reached a later stage in my fitness routine. During the initial period of improving fitness, the exercise becomes so tiring that you feel sleepy a few hours after the workout regime, robbing any time for intimacy. But when your schedule stabilizes and your body adapts to the exercise, you will see the above benefit.

But you will be curious to ask if a testosterone spike only lasts for a few minutes or for hours. So where does the benefit lie?

It is true that testosterone spikes are temporary, but that spike is very useful. There are numerous other health benefits too from working out. Flexibility in the body due to exercise and growth of many types of muscles, all play a role in enhancement of the sex life.

Are there exercises that can provide bigger boost to testosterone?

Yes, according to Todd Schroeder, PhD, University of Southern California, the following strategies will give you an even bigger boost in testosterone, which is backed of by research.

- Use more muscles. (For instance, a full-body workout affects this hormone more than doing one exercise, such as biceps curls.)
- Lift heavier weights rather than doing many repetitions with light weights.
- Have shorter rest periods during your workout.

Excess of everything is bad and the same is true for exercises also. According to a study done at the University of British Columbia and published in the *British Journal of Sports Medicine*, men who ran more than 40 miles per week had testosterone levels that were one-fifth lower than men who ran shorter distances. Research suggests that some exercises certainly reduce testosterone levels when overdone, for example, anyone doing long cardio programmes for prolonged jogging or marathon etc., can face this. People overdo to get quick results, which is the wrong approach to attain fitness.

> **Caution** Exercise breaks down your muscles; rest stimulates growth and repair. The combination of too much exercise with too little recovery time can result in testosterone reduction.

What are the signs of overtraining which you can watchout for?

According to Schroeder some of the signs are:

- **Excessive soreness:** Some soreness will always be there. So, don't stop exercising because of that. Focus on the word 'excessive'.
- **Trouble recovering from workouts:** Watch out for this as it depends from person to person. If in doubt, you must check with a general physician.
- **Trouble sleeping:** Trouble in sleeping could be due to many other reasons too. However, it could be associated with overtraining as well. Normally, exercise should aid in sleeping.
- **Losses in performance and strength:** This could also be due to improper diet so you must check with general physician, if the problem persists.

> **Caution** One should have sufficient rest between workouts and eat healthy food to enable the body to heal. Do not go for quick results as they will cause more damage over time.

Female Sex Hormones

Female sex hormones are estrogen and progesterone, which constantly keep changing. During the first two weeks of the menstrual cycle, hormones in a female's body are dominated by estrogen; the second two weeks where ovulation begins, progesterone takes over as the primary hormone, and this cycle repeats on a monthly basis.

But women also have testosterone, which are normally fifteen to twenty folds lower in concentration to that of the testosterone present in men. So, based on the fact that women's hormone levels vary, a study conducted by

The Applied Physiology Laboratory in the Department of Exercise and Sports Science at the University of North Carolina, aimed to examine the testosterone response to exercise in women under conditions of high and low estrogen levels. Results concluded that *it did not matter where women were in their menstrual cycle with respect to the degree of interaction with testosterone.* Though the same study also concluded that prolonged aerobic exercise induces short-term elevations in testosterone, which appears to be unrelated to estrogen levels and menstrual cycle phases.

So basically, when you workout, your body is either making more testosterone or destroying less of it. Either way, it is good to exercise for better testosterone. Though testosterone is not the primary sex hormone in women, but the optimal quantity, which is much less than men, is required for a healthy female body.

> **Tip!** It is not just men, women also need a balanced testosterone for female metabolic, sexual and muscular function. And just like men, it is important for women to have a healthy hormonal balance.

Now let us focus on the relationship between exercise and the changing hormonal level during menstrual cycle. A beautiful article 'Estrogen: Your New Training Partner' on oxygenmag.com in March 2014 suggests ways to deal with the exercise in such a changing environment in a women's cycle. Normally, one expects to feel and perform better for demanding workouts when estrogen is high and feel the worst during menstruation and when progesterone is at its peak during the late luteal phase and into the early follicular phase.

'While some women may have few noticeable effects during their cycle, others may notice fatigue, difficulty working out, cramping, bloating and increased perception of effort, particularly in the days leading up to and the first few days of their period,' says Dr Carolyn Smith in the article mentioned above.

'The fluctuations in estrogen and progesterone throughout your menstrual cycle alter the ability to build muscle and recover,' says Stacy Sims, PhD, exercise physiologist and co-founder of Osmo Nutrition (osmonutrition.com). It is natural and makes sense to take advantage of those peak estrogen-dominant days in the first half of the cycle to work on muscle tone. A study in the *International Journal of Sports Medicine* found that:

> Doing more weight training in the estrogen-dominant follicular phase and less training in the progesterone-dominant luteal phase led to greater strength gains in the quadriceps. Focus your hardest strength-training workouts when your estrogen is at its highest during the follicular phase—days 6 to 14. And best time for cardio for better result is days six to 20.

It does not mean that you should not exercise during the latter part of the cycle when progesterone is dominant. Progesterone is catabolic, which reduces the body's ability to recover and build muscle. However, during the days when a woman is menstruating, one may want to delay tough sessions at the gym. But for healthy living, exercise is a must irrespective of the stage of the cycle, and hormonal changes also vary based on age, fitness level and other parameters.

Women are more careful about their body fat. It is no secret that exercise can help lower fat levels in your body, but if the body fat percentage is too low, it is again bad for health. Women body fat percentage has to be generally higher than men for healthy living. In women, fat level and estrogen are related. Women who are gymnasts, athletes and models with extremely low body fat may have problems producing sufficient amounts of estrogen. Regular workouts for the non-athlete can aid estrogen levels and if you are overweight, you may be producing too much estrogen, and a regular exercise regime may help bring your levels down.

> **Caution** Beware of having lower body fat, which will lead to lower than required estrogen, which is bad for health.

Impact on Sex Life

For this topic, a research conducted in 1990 by White and colleagues at the University of California, San Diego, is often quoted even after decades. They had chosen two groups of men, with an average age of 48, who are healthy but mostly sedentary in nature. Both groups of men were assigned different sets of activities to be undertaken for 60 minutes a day. They were observed over a period of 9 months. One group of 17 men undertook walking at a moderate pace for around 4 days per week on an average. The other group of 78 people was asked to take up aerobic exercises for three and half days per week on an average. Each group maintained a daily diary of their exercises, diet, smoking and sexual activity during the first and last month of the programme.

An analysis of their diary entries revealed that the latter group who undertook aerobic exercises reported higher levels of sexual intimacy, more satisfying orgasms and more reliable sexual functioning. This proved that men who are physically active and engaged in aerobic exercises 3 or 4 days a week regularly, for at least an hour, have frequent and better sex. However, all men experienced some improvement, leading the researchers to conclude that enhanced sexuality is directly proportionate to their improvement in physical fitness.

Fitness Does Enhance Sex Life, But How?

NYC Certified fitness trainer Mike Giliotti said that it's the smaller muscles, which one can't see or feel, make the difference. Improved muscle tone can increase sexual satisfaction as science has proven that orgasm depends on multiple muscle activities. Not only for young men, but also for mature men, fitness improves the cardiovascular functioning, which then helps in improving sexual function.

> **Tip!** Fitness will help in enhancing the muscles big or small and help in improved cardiovascular functions, which can aid in improved sex life.

He further said in www.activetimes.com to try five sexercises to keep the sex life awesome. Though the following exercises are geared towards men, they also work great for women who want a boost to their sex life, as per Giliotti.

Push-ups

If you're going to pick just one exercise to engage yourself in, this is the one to go for. Do 3 sets of 12 to 15 repetitions.

Abdominals

Good old-fashioned crunches are good enough. Lie on your back, hands supporting your neck, knees bent and your feet on the floor. Then bring your body up just enough to get your shoulders off the ground. Do 3 to 5 sets of 15 to 20 repetitions.

Extra ab oomph

Giliotti suggested that both men and women should do bridges. Lying on your back, knees bent, feet on the floor, lift your hips up and down 15 times. Do 3 sets of 15 repetitions. Men can also try pelvic tilts. Standing up or lying down, straighten your lower back and pull your belly button in until your lower back touches the wall or floor. Women can try Kegels. Contract your pelvic muscles by tightly squeezing the muscles for 3 seconds and then relax for 3 seconds. Do 10 to 15 repetitions 3 times a day.

Deadlifts

This exercise will keep your back as strong as it can be and make your legs and torso workout. Deadlifts, in which you start in a neutral bent-over position and raise a weighted barbell or dumbbells from the ground, are easy to do and easy to do wrong with. So, technique is important to prevent injury.

Torso side bends and twists

Torso side bends and twists will keep your upper body strong and give you stamina. Gilliotti further suggested doing them on the cable crossover machine for maximum effect and pushing or pulling exercise in the gym. Rows, flyes and lateral raises on the cable crossover machine will do a great job of enhancing the performance in the bedroom.

Caution A trainer or someone knowledgeable enough should monitor all the above sex-enhancing exercises to ensure that one's body is capable of doing it.

A strong article was published in Caloilab.com, which, quite bluntly, was forcing the reader to take up fitness for a happy sexual life.

The article titled 'The Relationship between Fitness and Sex' written by one Dr J, a Surgeon from Florida and fitness freak. It states that 'abdominal fat is metabolically active. One of its activities is to change testosterone to estrogen. Excessive estrogen has a feminizing effect on males. The nuts and bolts of it all is that with this extra estrogen, the penis may shrink and not function sexually when you become obese. All the extra estrogen that is made and stored in fat will make Mr Happy go bye-bye. You can call it fat-related andropause if that sounds more medical. In addition, "it" may or may not come back if you lose the weight. Have you perhaps noticed this if you are overweight? Sure, you think it's the little bit of fat just covering it up a bit. Sorry—it may be going on a very long vacation. I know I'm hitting below the belt here, but I'm really disappointed with men not being in better shape.'

Let us shift the focus on women and the impact of fitness on their sexual life. There is hardly any brainer that women would not be different from men, and those who exercise frequently should have better sex life. Researchers at the University of Texas, Austin, found that 'female participants were 169 per cent more aroused (as indicated by blood flow in genital tissue) while watching a short porn flick after 20 minutes of vigorous cycling than when they watched it without riding beforehand. When you get excited, blood surges into the clitoral bulbs, making the entire region around the vagina responsive to pleasure. Cardiovascular exercise can help blood pump faster to the right parts of your body; it can also reduce chronic inflammation, which can damage blood vessels and decrease circulation, putting a damper on your sexual bliss.' It makes it amply clear that women who frequently exercise become aroused more quickly and can orgasm faster and more intensely.

Can Fitness Reduce Libido?

It could reduce the libido, if you are very tired from the exercises. In the initial days of joining the gym, exercises can cause fatigue and soreness, therefore reducing libido. But as you proceed towards achieving fitness, where muscles are well-toned and flexible, your sexual life is bound to improve.

Physical benefits

Since the induction into fitness, my annual comprehensive health check-up reports show all parameters within the normal range. Even though most of these ranges are being questioned in the latest studies, being within the permissible range gives me immense satisfaction.

> **Tip!** Fitness can correct many parameters in the blood-test report, and help to get rid of medicines taken to correct certain out-of-range parameters.

When I started going to the gym, my body reflexes were average. I used to be careful while bending and turning quickly to avoid a muscle pull. Now, I can smoothly do these movements without any concern.

When I was on the path to fitness, something else was

also happening to me; I cannot say whether it was to my advantage or not. I, who had only had verbal arguments with others and never a history of getting physically violent, was beginning to get aggressive. During arguments, my fist would automatically tighten. But thanks to my strong willpower, I never crossed the line. As hilarious as it may sound, I could actually have my way by just standing in an overtly aggressive posture, without uttering a word. My first such experience went somewhat like this:

One day, my driver had to suddenly pull the brakes of the car as the vehicle ahead of us had stopped abruptly. An autorickshaw, which was trying to avoid the inadvertent collision, hit the side of my car. I knew this was not my driver's fault, but knew what would happen the next moment and that is exactly what happened. My driver stopped the car at the side of the road and the autorickshaw driver did the same. My driver stepped out of the vehicle, and before he could speak, the aggressive autorickshaw driver started hurling abuses at him. My driver joined in and a few choice abuses were exchanged. The autorickshaw driver was accusing my driver of suddenly stopping the car, which caused damage to his vehicle. Instead of apologizing for hitting my car, he was asking for money to repair his vehicle. By then, other bystanders had begun to gather. I did not want to prolong the scene. I came out of my car, rolled up my sleeves and stared at the autorickshaw driver without uttering a word. I gestured asking my driver to shut up.

The argument stopped at once. The autorickshaw driver looked at me, I glared back at him and then looked at my car's bumper, which had a dent. I took a few steps towards him with a stern look, but kept quiet.

'Ok, you people can go; I will spend my money to repair

my vehicle,' the autorickshaw driver said to the crowd and my driver. He then went back to his vehicle and we did the same. My driver was super excited after the incident.

'It was entirely his fault and to top it all, he was asking for money from us. But sir, how did you manage without saying a single word! The way you were looking at him seemed so scary, as if you were going to hit him hard.'

'It's ok. But you should also maintain distance between the two vehicles while driving,' I replied.

I was surprised because so far I had never witnessed such an impact of my personality to win an argument without moving a finger. I now understood why some sports persons or those who are physically strong become aggressive at the slightest provocation or fall into trouble with fans and journalists. This might have been due to the level of fitness they have achieved.

> **Caution** Fitness increases self-confidence and triggers some aggressive behaviour initially until you adjust to the new normal. Ensure that you realize this change, control and avoid the aggression.

By now adjectives like 'strong', 'powerful', 'high testosterone', 'stud', 'alpha male', etc., have started to flow in. Such adjectives coming at this stage of my life and career are somewhat embarrassing. I cannot forget another incident that happened to me a few years back.

I had been calling my regular trainer to help me in one exercise. He was busy helping others and then got a phone call. When he finished his call, he came back and started chatting with another gym member. I was becoming impatient, went close to him and nudged on his strong arm with my fist. He was startled and looked at me holding his arm with his other hand.

'Oh sir! Do not do that. You are not the same anymore; you have a lot of energy now. Had you hit me hard, I could have dislocated my arm.'

For a moment, I was happy because that was the first time in my life someone said such a thing to me, but I suddenly realized that the person who I was becoming, was not me. I cannot possibly cause any physical harm to anyone.

This fitness also brought a new kind of responsibility to me—to keep the new-found high energy within myself. This phase did not last too long as my body adjusted quickly to this change, but one thing changed permanently. Unknowingly, I developed a habit of occasionally clenching one of my fists and hitting the other palm with it. This helped me in releasing some of my energy.

> **Tip!** Physical benefit of fitness is certainly immense. Flexibility, energy, posture and having a better body fat percentage are some of them.

Mental benefits

Other than physical benefits of fitness, there are the mental benefits too. Since childhood, we have been told that 'healthy mind resides in a healthy body'. In earlier sections, I have covered how the confidence of a person improves with fitness. Confidence is really an attractive thing. Fitness enhances self-esteem. These are basically the mental benefits one can get from fitness. In times where the role of the family in choosing a partner for a girl or a boy is diminishing at a fast rate and where it is up to the individual to look for his or her life partner, tell me who would want to go on a date with an underconfident person. Dr Michael Young of the University of Arkansas did a study with 408 graduate students (both male and female). The study revealed that mental benefits from working out were just as powerful as physical benefits if not more when it came to sexual satisfaction. Mental fitness which comes from self-confidence, high self-esteem and feeling good, together with physical fitness and job satisfaction is a deadly mix. Though I always try to be happy, this transformation is making my happiness infectious.

Let us see how exercise could help people recover from certain mental illness. While writing this section for the book, I took help of various articles. One of them is 'The Mental Benefits of Exercise' published in helpguide.org by Lawrence Robinson, Jeanne Segal, PhD, and Melinda Smith, MA and was written in January 2017.

Anxiety

I have interacted with many people across sections of the society, and some people are by nature more anxious than others. It is not due to an actual incident but the anticipation of something unwanted might happen. Ironically, the probability of such things happening is thin, but the mental space it occupies is quite large. Such people will always be nervous for any small activity, which is outside their normal routine. Sometimes, I wonder how they can spend such a long life by always being under pressure of some anxiety. Our time could be well spent in writing down the anxiety and seeing the probability of its happening, and making a mental plan on how to respond to it if it occurs. This should put to rest most of our simple anxieties, but it is not as simple as it sounds. Sometimes I too fall into the anxious mode, but then I try to come out of it quickly by applying the above approach. One other thing, which also helps me, is to talk about my anxiety with someone whom I trust. It is better if that person is able to give some sound advice. There is a caveat here. My observation is that most of the time what we speak about is not the actual issue, but we confuse the symptoms with the root cause. So, taking external advice could be beneficial if the root cause is understood better, else just having a patient listener is good enough.

Helpguide.org article states that:

> Exercise is a natural and effective anti-anxiety treatment. It relieves tension and stress, boosts physical and mental energy, and enhances well-being through the release of endorphins. Anything that gets you moving can help, but you'll get a bigger benefit if you pay attention instead of zoning out. For example, try to notice the sensation of your feet hitting the ground, or the rhythm of your breathing, or the feeling of the wind on your skin. By adding this mindfulness element—really focusing on your body and how it feels as you exercise—you'll not only improve your physical condition faster, but you may also be able to interrupt the flow of constant worries running through your head.

Tip! Constant flow of worry gets disrupted by exercise not only due to release of endorphins, but also the focus will shift on breathing, posture, count and focus on the body part on which the exercise is targeted.

Depression

Depression could be due to any reason. It could be one or a mix of many things causing it. Your job, family, perceived sense of not doing good in life, not living up to the expectation of those who matter, and so on. However, poor health could be an important cause of depression too.

In the webMD.com article 'Exercise and Depression', it says:

> Many studies show that people who *exercise* regularly benefit with a positive boost in mood and lower rates of *depression*. Improved self-esteem is a key psychological benefit of regular *physical activity*. When you exercise, your body releases chemicals called endorphins. These endorphins interact with the receptors in your *brain* that reduce your perception of pain. Endorphins also trigger a positive feeling in the body, similar to that of *morphine*. For example, the feeling that follows a run or workout is often described as "euphoric". That feeling, known as a "runner's high", can be accompanied by a positive and energizing outlook on life. Endorphins act as analgesics, which means they diminish the perception of pain. They also act as sedatives. They are manufactured in your *brain*, spinal cord, and many other parts of your body and are released in response to *brain* chemicals called neurotransmitters. The neuron receptors endorphins bind to are the same ones that bind some pain medicines. However, unlike with morphine, the activation of these receptors by the body's endorphins does not lead to *addiction* or dependence.

In March 2014, Olga Khazan wrote an article 'For Depression, Prescribing Exercise Before Medication' in *The Atlantic* mentioning that 'depression affects 25 per cent of Americans.' She added that 'the use of antidepressants has increased 400 per cent between 1988 and 2008. They're now one of the three most-prescribed categories of drugs, coming in right after painkillers and cholesterol medications'.

After 15 years of research on the depression-relieving effects of exercise, she asks why are there still so many people on pills in the article? She concluded by saying, 'Either the doctor is not savvy or patients are looking for a quick fix, and resist taking *physical action* to improve their own situation'.

> **Tip!** Doctors are being advised to prescribe exercise rather than anti depressant for patients suffering from depression.

Stress

In our professional world, we use the word stress loosely. Work overload is sometimes called stress. Not being able to handle a difficult stakeholder like the manager at work can cause stress. If someone is unable to find a solution to a problem or is unable to finish work within the expected time frame can also cause stress. The meaning of stress in the Oxford Dictionary is: 'State of mental or emotional strain or tension resulting from adverse or demanding circumstances.' In a nutshell, stress is basically what you feel.

If two people are assigned the same problem to tackle independently, will the level of stress for both be the same? The answer is simply 'no'. It is basically how you receive the problem, and how equipped you are to handle it. So, stress is not dependent on the source of the problem, it is purely on how you take it.

Stress does not always have to have a negative impact; it could also have a positive one. Some types of stresses can improve performance and make people realize their potential and capability. Stress could happen in any sphere, it could be personal, social, professional or anything else.

What happens when you are stressed?

The same helpguide.org article states,

> Ever noticed how your body feels when you're under stress? Your muscles may be tense, especially in your face, neck, and shoulders, leaving you with back or neck pain, or painful headaches. You may feel tightness in your chest, a pounding pulse, or muscle cramps. You may also experience problems such as insomnia, heartburn, stomachache, diarrhea, or frequent urination. The worry and discomfort of all these physical symptoms can in turn lead to even more stress, creating a vicious cycle between your mind and body. Exercising is an effective way to break this cycle. As well as releasing endorphins in the brain, physical activity helps to relax the muscles and relieve tension in the body. Since the body and mind are so closely linked, when your body feels better so, too, will your mind.

Tip! Exercise relaxes the muscle, relieves the tension. As your body feels better, and mind and body being interconnected, mind will feel better thereby reducing the stress.

Benefits of exercise run deep into our brain. A well-known fact is that we are full of energy when our heart functions well, we experience sound sleep and have a higher self-confidence.

> **Caution** One can get mental benefit from exercise rather than resorting to alcohol or drugs.

So, the question arises: Is it is harder to do exercise for mental benefits? Helpguide.org article suggests that one can reap all the physical and mental benefits with 30 minutes of moderate exercise five times a week. Even two 15-minute or three 10-minute exercises per day is also fine. This means that some kind of activity will always be better than doing none.

I had mentioned earlier that I used to do brisk walking regularly, but over the years it started giving diminishing returns. So, following a moderate exercise routine is good to start with. However, if you want to be fit, you must undertake more than moderate exercises where the heart rate rises to the threshold limit, depending upon your age and fitness level, to experience the benefits.

I am enjoying all the benefits with the increased fitness level, which in turn is making me happy. This has been noticed not only by my team in India but also by others upon my visit to the offices situated at different geographical locations. One of the employees, who has worked with me for around a decade, was discussing a critical issue with me. The issue was somewhat tricky and I was glad that we resolved it. Just before leaving, he stopped at the door turned around and said:

'You have changed.'

I was surprised at his statement.

'Sorry, what did you say?' I asked.

'You have started smiling a lot, your anger has reduced, and you have more patience. This makes me feel more welcome to discuss and share everything with you. Earlier I used to be frightened of you in such tricky situations,' he said.

People associate a typical profile for the role that I have in office. Over the years, that stereotype image that people have in mind has changed. Some of the new comers in the office ask their peers if I am the same person on this job. One day, an employee met me in the corridor of the office and I asked about the status of a critical programme which he was driving. While walking along he mentioned that he was undertaking kick-boxing and marathon running as his hobby and we briefly discussed the benefits of fitness. Suddenly, he asked:

'I think impact of fitness is more visible with the age. The gap widens between a fit person and a non-fit person as the age progresses, do you agree?'

'Why? Nowadays, diseases can happen at any age. With today's lifestyle and food habits, people can go out of shape at any age,' I replied.

'Yes, but when my father and some of my relatives were at your age, I could see wrinkles, sagging skin and dark circles,' he continued.

'Your job is more stressful and round the clock. But still, the energy, freshness and positivity which you spread is much higher than what my father exhibited at his age, whereas his responsibility and stress was lesser,' he finished his statement.

This sums up the immense benefits which fitness provides.

SPECIAL SECTION #5

Fitness Tips for Women

SHWETA MEHTA

Techie turned Fitness Athlete, Winner of MTV Roadies 2017 and Jerai Classic Women's Physique 2016. Represented India in Asian Championship

Weight training has been a men's sport, but women mostly spend hours doing cardiovascular exercises in the name of fitness training. Fact is though cardio is important for keeping a good heart, but one will never get the desired results by only doing cardiovascular activities.

Let me straight get on to myths related to women's fitness:

Myth #1: Weight Training Will Make Women Bulky

Women are scared of the word 'muscles'. The moment they hear about it they start forming an image of a big muscular man. They become insecure and afraid of lifting weights. Testosterone is the main cause of muscle building. A woman's body doesn't have equal or even come close to the amount of testosterone which a man's body has. That's why lifting weights will never make a woman's body muscular. The reality is that weight-lifting will make women's body slimmer by toning the muscles.

Myth #2: Long Hours of Cardiovascular Exercises Will Help Losing Weight

Weight training will not only help you lose fat faster or burn calories faster but will also help you in overall health. By only doing cardio exercises, one will lose muscle mass along with fat. Muscles are important, because a body, which does not have enough muscles will invite more fat deposit. Less muscle means lower metabolism. So it is important to do weight training to develop muscle which in turn will help in weight loss.

Myth #3: More the Workout, More the Weight Loss; More One Eats, More the Weight Gain

Diet plays a major role in gaining or losing weight. First of all, you should know how many calories you are burning in your day to day life, and then figure out how many more you need to burn. Second, you need to find out a proper diet plan as per your calorie intake. There are various types of diet plans available, but basics of gaining and losing weight remains the same. Gaining weight requires calorie surplus and losing weight on the other hand requires calorie deficit. Calorie surplus is a state in which you consume more calories than you burn.

Myth #4: Do Unlimited Crunches to Reduce Belly Fat And to Get Six Packs

Fat deposits in women are mostly on their thighs, lower abdomen and arms, but there is no spot reduction. It is physically impossible to focus on fat cells of a particular body part. When you workout, the body fat from the entire body drops and not from any specific body part. Concentrating more on compound exercises and not just crunches alone will make one lose that belly fat.

Myth #5: One Cannot Lift After the Age of 40

You can improve strength at any age, though it gets challenging with age and takes more time. Anyone can get the result provided the person is dedicated to the journey of fitness. Needless to say that workout has to be done with right training methods and accompanied with proper nutritious meals.

Myth #6: Once One Stops Weight Training, One Will Gain More Weight Than Before

It is all about calorie intake. Workout helps in burning the calories so even if you are eating well, workout is burning the calories. When you stop the exercise, normally people do not reduce their calorie intake and continue to eat the same or more. Thus, calorie intake becomes more than what your body needs, causing weight gain.

Now, let us see how lifting weights can be helpful:

- **Reduction in Osteoporosis:** After you finish the weight training, your body needs additional oxygen and your body continues to burn calories. This physiological effect is called excess post-exercise oxygen consumption, or EPOC. It prevents osteoporosis. As per International Osteoporosis Foundation (IOF), worldwide, one in three women above the age of 50 experiences osteoporosis fractures. Strength training over a period of time can help in increasing the spinal bone density.
- **Reduction in Diabetes:** It reduces the risk of diabetes and increases the consumption of glucose.
- **Reduction in Cardiovascular Disease:** It increases HDL, reduces LOL and it lowers the risk of cardiovascular diseases.

Workout during Menstrual Cycle

Training in the first two weeks, starting from your menstrual cycle is the best time for strength and resistance training and for HIIT. Your body can perform the best and ideally, you can push more these days.

Working out reduces the level of stress and anxiety; it also treats headache and irregular flow. However, it is okay to take a break of a day or two and listen to your body if you are not feeling like working out. If you are excessively low and skipping the workout, then go for a walk, pamper yourself. Do not take this as an excuse and keep on relaxing for a week. As you will have to face this every month, you cannot afford losing one week every month with such an excuse. As you know your body well, the more you will observe your body, the more you will educate yourself to adjust the exercises accordingly. Yes, you can train during menstrual cycle.

Workout Routine

You can do bodyweight training even if you do not have access to gym. You can perform resistance training in the gym with the help of machines or at home. Here are a few important exercises and their benefits, which you can perform for 50-60 minutes anywhere and anytime.

Push-ups: Push-up is the greatest exercise of all. It's a compound exercise, which means it involves various muscle groups at once. It's the best full body workout. You can begin with keeping knees on the ground and later once you perfect the push-ups, you can try other variations of this exercise such as pike diamond push-ups, clap push-ups, superman push-ups, etc., to increase the intensity of your workout. Repetition range: 10-15, three sets.

Pull-ups: Pull-ups is another upper body compound exercise. It is a very efficient exercise, because at each repetition your entire upper body, shoulders, arms, forearms, upper back and lower back are involved. Repetition range: 6-8, 3 sets.

Plank: This is an overall strength building exercise, which works on various muscles, hence improves posture and balance. It is one vital exercise for abdominal muscles. It engages all the major core muscles, including abdomen and obliquus. So do you need those six packs? Start mastering the plank. Hold for 45-60 seconds, 3 sets.

Squats: Squat is the king of exercises. This is another lower body compound exercise. Since it is a functional exercise, it plays an important role in real-life activities. Squat has many variations: close stance squat, wide stance squat, sumo squat, split squat, etc. You can perform all of them without additional weight and still see good results. Repetition range: 15-20, 3-4 sets.

Lunges: You don't like them? Well, you can't escape them. Lunges are another brilliant exercise for the lower body; it mainly targets the quadriceps, but also engages other big muscles like glutes and hamstrings. It's a unilateral functional exercise which directly improves your real life tasks. You have to put extra effort to keep your upper body straight which results in better core stability. Front lunges and backward lunges are the generic ones. Repetition range: 10-12 each leg, 3 sets.

Burpee: This is definitely the No. 1 exercise to burn fat. This full body explosive exercise not only helps in building strength, but burns lots of calories. So you can give a break to treadmill. Burpee exercise can be modified according to your convenience. You can keep it easy by not performing push-ups, and you can also make it difficult by adding a tough variation of push-ups. Repetition range: 10-15, 3 sets.

Squat jumps: This is a vital aerobic exercise for leg strength. Like burpees, this also helps in burning calories at a faster rate. And, by the way, if you are looking for those toned legs this is for you. Similarly, there is lunge jump, which is a little difficult than squat jump, you can first master squat jump before you start lunge jumps. Repetition range: 12-15, 3 sets.

Mountain climbers: This is a complete abdominal and cardio exercise which helps you to cut belly fat. Leave crunches for a while and try mountain climbers for that flat tummy. Another variation of mountain climber can be grasshopper. Repetition range: 25-30 each leg, 3 sets.

Superman/prone back extension: Lower back strengthening is very important for women, and superman serves as the best exercise for that. If done regularly, you can get relief from your back pain. Also incorporating this exercise in squat workout session will make it a complete leg workout, because it works on glutes and hamstrings. You can also alternate superman exercise with cat and camel stretches. Repetition range: 20–25, 3 sets.

Bridge: This mainly works on glutes and hamstrings. Glutes is a power house for any explosive exercise or a sprint. Strengthening glutes helps you perform such exercises better and improves athletic performance. You can try variations like single leg bridge, weighted bridge, bridge pulses, etc., to add intensity to your workout. Repetition range: 15–20, 4 sets.

Diet and Its Impact on Fitness

Diet, a clean and balanced diet will do half of the job for you. No matter how hard you are working out in the gym, if you are not eating clean you will never get the desired result. Let us look into some misconceptions in your diet.

Are juices good for health? You think juices are good and that is why you are on liquid diet. You wonder you are still not getting any desired results.

Yes, fruits are healthy but in a limited quantity. A glass of juice will have at least six times the servings mentioned in it, packed with sugar. Such a high dose of sugar is hindering the result. Stick to a high-protein diet with limited quantity of fruits and nuts. Also, a smoothie is much better than juice. A smoothie contains fibre and the peels of fruits.

Are you drinking less water to avoid water retention? This is another big mistake most people commit by consuming less water to avoid water retention. You should drink at least 3–4 litres of water a day. Drinking enough water helps in overall body functionality by keeping you hydrated.

Is salt bad as it makes you feel bloated? You should consume normal amount (in general, 1,500–2,000 mg) of salt every day and drink lots of water together so that body should not retain excessive sodium. Salt is important if taken in moderate quantities to balance electrolytes in the body.

Should you go for very low carbohydrate diet? Cutting carbs completely from your diet would not make you lose weight. Weight is lost due to calorie deficit in your diet, as mentioned earlier. Carbs provide fuel to your body. When you cut carbs from your diet you will see weight loss, but that is glycogen loss resulting into water loss. This is not good. You should plan for a balanced diet with moderate amount of carbs and less amount of fat with high-protein food.

Are you skipping food to consume fewer calories? It is a very big and common mistake people commit to achieve weight loss. You need to eat clean food and not junk and processed food to lower your calorie intake. You should control your portions on intake but do not skip any meal. Skipping meals will also slow down your metabolism which is not good for your body.

Your body and you have to work to maintain it. No one can help you get the desired results but you. Self-motivation is the key. You do not have to workout only to look good or compete, but workout to improve your health and to stay confident.

EIGHT

Exercise and Its Relationship with Injuries, Sickness and Jet Lag

What do we do when we injure ourselves during a fitness regime? Do exercises help even when we are sick? When professionals are on the move, how can they overcome a jet lag? Let us explore each of these queries.

Injuries

Just like sports, when we take up any kind of exercises we are prone to injuries. I experienced muscle strains during the initial few months of training at the gym. Since then, I have not experienced any injury and I have completed six years. I remind myself every day that the knee, neck and lower back must be protected. I avoided overdoing the exercises and more so, for the body parts which are prone to injuries. I was fine with the results taking longer to show. A proper warm up is always recommended before any exercise. After completing a workout regime, stretches to ease sore muscles, especially for the calves, hamstrings and lower back are very important. If some exercises are uncomfortable or if you think that they might cause injuries, you must ask your trainer or buddy or read about it on the Internet and decide accordingly. Normally, trainers can help you recover from minor pulls and injuries at the gym by suggesting stretches specific to the injury. They can also advice to avoid certain exercises if you already have some complications. If you are suffering from something serious, you must consult your general physician.

Amy Levin-Epstein's article 'Five Most Common Gym Injuries ' in www.mensfitness.com quotes personal trainer Justin Price, MA, who owns The BioMechanics Method, a corrective exercise and functional fitness facility in San Diego. According to Price, there are two main reasons for workout-related injuries. The first is poor posture during the day, which eventually weakens your entire musculoskeletal structure. To combat this, make sure your computer screen is positioned in a way that you do not have to strain or hunch to look at it. The other mistake is trying to do too much too fast, in both repetitions and weight. 'The problem that got you into the gym didn't happen overnight, so you can't undo it overnight,' says Price.

> **Tip!** Sedentary habits leading to wrong posture should be corrected. Patience in achieving the fitness can help in preventing an injury.

In the article, Price further states the most frequent injuries and its causes and preventions, which are mentioned below.

a) **Foot and ankle**
   Cause: 'People spend their days in front of their computers with rounded shoulders. When your shoulders are rounded, and you stand up, your weight falls to the front of your foot,' says Price. Take that misplaced

center of gravity and put it into running shoes, which naturally tip you forward with a heel higher than the toe, and your feet and ankles start to bear the brunt of any impact.

Prevention: 'You should look for a running shoe that isn't too high in the heel, or try a walking shoe, cross trainer or tennis shoe,' suggests Price. This will help spread the impact to the whole foot, you'll prevent problems like plantar fasciitis, achilles tendonitis, anterior compartment syndrome (a compression in the front of the ankle), lateral compression syndrome (a compression at the side of the ankle) and bunions.

b) **Knee**

Cause: 'We don't use our hip muscles during the day. Then we decide to go kickbox or do boot camp' says Price. The result is injury to the knee? 'If our feet aren't stable, due to improper footwear, and our hip muscles aren't strong, the knee gets all the stress,' says Price, who says that leg extensions, curls and presses don't help resolve the problem, because they don't strengthen the muscles of the feet and hips.

Prevention: 'A better exercise would be lunges. With a lunge, your hip and ankle are bending together, stabilizing and strengthening the knee,' says Price. To get even more benefit, do lunges both forwards and backwards, then side to side.

c) **Lower back**

Cause: 'If someone is rounded throughout the day in their upper back, and then they go to the gym and do an overhead shoulder lift standing, their upper back cannot extend properly. They straighten and arch upward from their lower back, which has a nervous breakdown [anything from soreness to more permanent injury] because it's getting all the stress,' says Price.

Prevention: Remember to stretch and strengthen your upper back to compensate for all the hunching you do at the office. Price suggests super-setting in straight-armed wall squats with the rest of your lifting regimen. 'Sit against a wall. Flatten your lower back into the wall, by tilting your pelvis under you. Straighten your arms in front of you, and try to raise arms up to your ears, without letting a gap form behind your lower back,' says Price. And whenever you can, exercise standing up. Really, you've sat enough at the office, right? 'Standing helps you engage bigger muscles in your body,' says Price.

d) **Shoulder**
Cause: If you haven't been convinced to hang up your mouse and pick up a hard hat, this just might do it. That carpal tunnel you're complaining about 9–5 could contribute to a gym injury after-hours. 'Your arms have to internally rotate when you type, which puts pressure on the shoulders,' says Price. 'Then you go to the gym and do chest press, shoulder press, push-ups, all also with your arms rotated in,' he notes. The outcome? Supraspinatus tendonitis—an overuse injury of the rotator cuff.

Prevention: You need to externally rotate your arms to balance your shoulders, and a great way to do that is by rowing with cables. 'Grab the cables in front of you and pull the arms back, rotating your palms away from you and behind you,' says Price.

e) **Neck**

   Cause: The other four areas being out of whack lead to a misalignment in your neck, says Price. 'If you sit with rounded shoulders, your neck follows your upper back, but then your eyes need to look at the screen, so you arch your neck and you get pain,' says Price. As if work wasn't a pain in the neck enough, you get to the gym and that poor posture follows you all the way to the bench press, where the real trouble starts, when you're lying on the bench but your back isn't flush with the pad. 'A lack of mobility and extension in your upper back will put stress on your lower back and neck,' says Price.

   Prevention: Clearly, when doing the bench press, make sure your lower back and neck are supported properly. Then, avoid putting additional stress on your neck with exercises that cause you to raise your arms over your head, especially if you've just put in a 12-hour day. Finally, strengthen your mid and upper back and improve your posture by doing reverse shrugs. 'Sit at the lat pull down. Grab the bar in front of you and do straight-arm pull downs. Pull down just the shoulder blades—not the arms—and go just slightly in front of you for three to four inches,' says Price. You'll feel it in your lower traps—which, once strong, will help you maintain your posture—and health—whether you're at the office or at the gym.

> **Caution** Listen to your body and if it is unreasonably uncomfortable don't do that exercise. If the problem persists, consult your doctor.

Exercise during Sickness

One question which is normally asked is: If I am sick shall I go to the gym or do any other fitness activity? This is a tricky question because it all depends upon what type of sickness you have. As I said in my earlier chapter, when I was having serious muscle pull in my upper body, my trainer asked me to continue the exercise but to focus on lower body. When my legs went stiff, he asked me to continue the exercise but to focus on my upper body. First, listen to your body. Your body will tell you whether you should do the exercise or not. Which type of exercise, how much exercise and when to stop during sickness could also be determined by discussing with your trainer, buddy or someone who is more knowledgeable at the gym, depending upon the signals given by your body. But the most crucial point is to be honest to yourself.

> **Caution** Do not tell the brain that one is feeling unwell and hence one will skip the exercise, when the actual reason is not any illness but simply laziness or fatigue.

In the initial period, this urge to bunk happened to me too for a good number of times. It was sometimes due to laziness, and at others due to tiredness. Whenever such feelings occurred, I ignored them and went to the gym. To my surprise, I have noticed many times that after the initial few minutes on the treadmill, I started to feel better and got motivated to continue.

Now as far as sickness is concerned, there are general illnesses like cold, cough, headache, etc.

> **Tip!** As a thumb rule during any sickness above the neck, one can go to gym, but any problem below the neck, it depends upon the specific sickness.

As said earlier, when in doubt always consult your general physician. Dennis Mann wrote an article 'Exercising when sick: a good move?' on webMD.com. He quoted Neil Schachter, MD, medical director of respiratory care at the Mount Sinai Medical Center in New York. 'If your symptoms are above the neck, including a *sore throat*, nasal congestion, *sneezing*, and *tearing eyes*, then it's OK to exercise,' Neil says. 'If your symptoms are below the neck, such as *coughing*, body aches, fever and *fatigue*, then it's time to hang up the running shoes until these symptoms subside.'

The article says very categorically that during fever, exercise is forbidden. The danger is that you can feel even sicker as exercise will raise the body temperature further. Most people who are fit tend to feel worse if they stop their exercise, but if you have a bad case of *flu* and can't even lift your head off the pillow, the question of exercising does not arise.

I follow the 'above the neck' and 'below the neck' rule while deciding about whether I should go to gym or not. However, the type of sickness or feeling uncomfortable has many hues, so when in doubt I do check with my trainer or ask a few other people. If doubt persists, I consult my general physician.

> **Caution** If one is under any medication, it is important to check with the general physician about exercising. Probably, you could exercise after the medication but only after a few hours or so.

Those who are addicted to exercising like me, skipping due to sickness is quite depressing, but then one should follow what the general physician advises. Maybe you can undertake a simple walk instead of doing treadmill. If no exercise is possible, think positive, take rest and feel happy.

Jet Lag

Crossing multiple time zones during air travel makes people dysfunctional for a good number of days. Based on my experience and information gathered from talking with other professionals, it gets worse with age. It could take anytime from a few days to few weeks to get over it and varies from person to person. Some folks take medicines to beat the jet lag. I have never tried any medicine.

I tried to cope up with jet lag in the following two steps: First, I try to slowly set my sleeping pattern and biological clock to the destination time zone a few days before the journey. Normally, I travel to the West Coast of the USA, which is around 12 hours behind my home time. So trying to adjust with a 12-hour cycle is easier for me. Trying is important even if you may not succeed. If you cannot sleep at least try to take a nap. You can also try to align sleep time with the destination's night time during your flight. Some people are unable to sleep in the flight, at least they should try to nap or close their eyes and listen to some soothing music. Use an eye patch to get sleep. Those who get sleep in the flight consider themselves lucky.

> **Tip!** To get sleep in the flight, you need to tire the body before you fly. A well-rested body before flying will make sleeping difficult in the flight.

Second, I choose my travel itinerary in such a way so that I reach the destination in the broad daylight. This enables me to have daylight while landing and get my eyes adjusted it.

> **Tip!** The exposure to sunlight helps in reducing the jet lag effect.

If I am reaching the destination on a working day, or even as late as afternoon, I try to attend office even if for a few hours or remain outside the hotel. If reaching on the weekend, I try to go out rather than stay in the hotel during daytime. By being away from bed and busy in some activity helps in avoiding the sleep at odd hours and thereby overcoming the jet lag.

One more thing which I have noticed is that I can cope with jet lag faster if I travel in economy class rather than business class. In the economy class, my sleep will not be deep and long due to discomfort. But when I travel in business class the comfort prolongs my sleep or makes the body very well rested. As said earlier, the body has to get tired to be able to sleep, so it is easier to beat jet lag while travelling in economy class. Business class provides comfort and thereby makes attending office easier on the day of arrival but getting sleep in the night will be difficult.

For the next few days at the destination city, I try to hit the gym or do some exercise in the morning time because sometimes jet lag does not affect the first day but hits you on the second day or the third day and so on. When I return, as most of the international flights land late at night or early morning in India, I try to reach on weekdays, so that I can attend office in the day and hit the gym in the evening at my usual time.

> **Caution** Jet lag is more difficult when one travels against time that is from west to east.

I observed that it takes more time and challenge to beat the jet lag when I return home and I initially thought that it might be because it is home but when my colleagues in the west also mentioned that it is more challenging for them adjusting to the time in India, rather than back home. So, I searched for an answer and got a scientific one.

'Most of our internal clocks are a little bit slow, and in the absence of consistent light cues—like when you travel across time zones—the pacemaker cells in your body want to have a longer day,' said Michelle Girvan, a physicist at the University of Maryland, in the article 'Why Jet Lag Can Feel Worse When You Travel from West to East' written by Joanna Klein in *The New York Times*.

'This is all because the body's internal clock has a natural period of slightly longer than 24 hours, which means that it has an easier time travelling west and lengthening the day than travelling east and shortening the day,' Dr. Girvan said.

John Donnelly's article 'Running Away from Jet Lag: How Exercise Can Help Overcome Travel Fatigue' in *The Washington Post* in April 2013 beautifully captures four actions one should do to overcome jet lag. According to him:

> One is getting sleep on the plane. (It's more important than watching that second movie.) A second is not drinking alcohol during a flight—a lesson learned only in recent years; it's the best way to avoid feeling lousy when you land. A third is to go to bed in your destination at a normal bedtime. But the fourth is the most important: Run the next morning. Lots of studies

have made clear the important health benefits of regular exercise. But research also suggests that exercise helps with time-change adjustments and may speed up the return to normal circadian rhythms, or the internal body clock.

A 1987 study found that *hamsters* that ran on an exercise wheel adjusted to a new lab-created time zone in a day and a half, on average, while those that did no exercise took more than eight days to adjust.

So, following all of the above advice will certainly help in overcoming jet lag and fitness plays a key role in this.

SPECIAL SECTION #6

Maintaining Fitness in the Office

DR GOPAKUMAR
*Founder & CEO of Core Physio India and
Certified physio and sports trainer*

These days, it seems like everyone is working more hours and using the old 'no-time-to-exercise' excuse more than ever. But what if you could actually workout at work? Stretching is one part of a successful ergonomics programme that can help to prevent musculoskeletal disorders, pain and discomfort. Stretching allows your body time to recover, relax and prepare for the next session. Frequent stretching will also help prevent muscles from getting stiff and reduce discomfort. You don't need to go for a long run to get your daily dose of cardio. Heart-pumping routine you can do anywhere, even while you're at work.

Let us look into the type of medical conditions which are being observed in professionals due to their lack of maintaining sufficient exercise and keeping right posture at the workplace.

Organ Damages

- **Heart**: When you sit, blood flows slower and muscles burn less fat, which makes it easier for fatty acids to clog your heart.
- **Pancreas**: Your body's ability to respond to insulin is affected by just one

day of excess sitting, which leads your pancreas to produce increased amounts of insulin, and this may lead to diabetes.
- **Digestion**: Sitting down after you've eaten causes your abdominal contents to compress, slowing down digestion.

Brain Damages

- Your brain function slows down when your body is sedentary for too long. Your brain will get less fresh blood and oxygen, which are needed to trigger the release of brain- and mood-enhancing chemicals.

Posture Problems

- **Strained Neck and Shoulders**: It's common to hold your neck and head forward while working at a computer or cradling a phone to your ear. This can lead to strains to your cervical vertebrae along with permanent imbalances, which can lead to neck strain, sore shoulders and back.
- **Back Problems**: Sitting puts more pressure on your spine than standing, and the toll on your back will get worse if you sit hunched in front of a computer.

Muscle Degeneration

- **Abdominal Problems:** Standing requires you to tense your abdominal muscles, which go unused when you sit, ultimately leading to weak abdominals.
- **Hip Problems**: Your hips also suffer from prolonged sitting, becoming tight and limited in range of motion because they are rarely extended. In the elderly, decreased hip mobility is a leading cause of falls.

Leg Disorders

- **Varicose Veins**: Sitting leads to poor circulation in your legs, which can cause swelling in your ankles, varicose veins and blood clots known as deep vein thrombosis (DVT).

- **Weak Bones**: Walking, running and engaging in other weight-bearing activities lead to stronger, denser bones. Lack of activity may cause weak bones and even osteoporosis.

Exercises at Your Office Desk

Let us look into this 10-minute exercise that can be performed at your desk easily.

- **Chair Dips (10 reps):** With your legs out in front of you, grab the edge of a chair (or desk) and lift yourself off the chair, lower your body downwards and lift it back up. At the end, you'll be conveniently back in your seat. Repeat it every hour; please be careful if your chair has wheels.
- **Book Press (10 reps):** Grab the heaviest book you have, hold it behind your head, and then extend your arms up. Drop it back down by your neck and repeat. Repeat it every hour. This is basically replacing dumbbells with the heavy book.
- **Triceps Desk Dips (10 reps):** Face yourself away from the desk, place hands shoulder-width apart with legs extended. Bend your arms, and then straighten to keep tension on your triceps and off your elbow joints. Before doing this exercise, please make sure your desk is stable and sturdy.
- **Tapping Toe (10 reps):** Tap your toe speedily on the floor under your desk. Repeat it every 30 minutes. Please make sure it does not make noise to distract others.
- **Leg Raise (10 reps):** Sit on your chair with leg down to form 90 degree with your body. Raise one leg, bring it down and keep it straight without bending your knees. After 10 reps repeat the same with your other leg. If possible, repeat it every hour.
- **Wrist Rotate (10 reps):** Rotate your wrists clockwise—10 reps—and anticlockwise—10 reps—for one hand, and then repeat the same for the other. Repeat it every 30 minutes.

- **Taking Stairs:** Avoid the elevator and take the stairs; it will help your heart to function well.

    Such exercises will help maintain a good fitness at work, but I would suggest that you do them at least a couple of times in a day. Maybe you can set an alert in your phone or on your calendar. And don't forget to drink sufficient amount of water at regular intervals.

Ergonomics at Your Workplace

We forget to ensure that we are using our chair, computer screen, mouse, keyboard and all other paraphernalia in a right way by maintaining a right posture. Here are some tips to have a comfortable workstation:

- Move the chair close to the workstation.
- Sit upright, supported by the chair's back support.
- Incline the seat 5–10° downwards.
- Sit with feet flat on the floor, or supported by a footstool.
- Some people like to sit in a slightly reclined position because it puts less stress on the back, although this may increase stress on the shoulders and neck when you reach for items. Supports your lower back and has adjustable armrests that allow your elbows to stay close to your sides. If you are not comfortable with armrests, move them out of your way. It is still important to keep your arms close to your sides even if you choose not to use armrests.
- Has a breathable, padded seat and rolls on five wheels for easy movement without tipping.
- Sit directly in front of the computer screen and keyboard to avoid neck twisting.
- Position screens at eye level (laptops should be raised and use a separate keyboard) and look into the far distance every few minutes to vary focal length and avoid eyestrain.
- Check the direction of the light source to avoid glare or reflections on the screen. Place the screen at right angles to the window when

possible. Apply a good quality glare filter on the monitor.
- Relax shoulders, periodically check they do not become tense, rise up or hunch.
- Let upper arms hang down naturally from shoulders; there should be a right angle at your elbow when typing.
- Never use keyboard or mouse wrist rests for permanently resting your wrists on while you are working.
- Your keyboard should be at a height that allows your elbows to be bent about 90 degrees and close to your sides.
- There are many variations for keyboard design, including split, curved, or rotated keyboards. Studies have not proved that these reduce injuries. But some people find them to be more comfortable. If you notice hand, arm or neck discomfort, your employer may have different keyboard styles for you to try. Different people find different styles work best for them.
- Many keyboards and keyboard trays have wrist supports to help keep your wrists in a neutral, almost straight position. But wrist pads are just there for brief rests. They are not meant to be used while you are typing. But some people find them helpful even during keying. When you type, try raising your wrists from the support so your wrists are in a neutral position. You may want to alternate between resting your wrists on the supports and raising them up.
- You can adjust the tilt of the keyboard. Some people find it more comfortable if the keyboard is flat or tilted slightly down at the top. Try different tilt angles to see what is most comfortable for you.

Workouts during Office Breaks

It might sound funny, but yes, you can do certain exercises inside the office too. Better to form a small group of people and if your office has a gym, go during break and try some mild floor exercise (to avoid changing the clothes), or if you can do it in the morning or evening with a little more exercise then you can carry fitness attire to change into.

- Do squats for 30 seconds and then hold that squat nice and low for 30 seconds. Repeat three times. Make sure you're keeping the weight on your heels and are sending the booty/hips back, not the knees forward. Knees shouldn't stick out farther than your toes. You can do these over a chair, tapping your butt to the seat each time and then holding a hover over it; or, just air squat.
- Do push-ups for 30 seconds and then triceps dips for 30 seconds. Repeat three times. For the push-ups, you can either do them on the floor, or at an angle. If you do them at an angle with hands on a platform (chair, desk, etc.) and feet on the floor, they'll be easier. If you do them at an angle with feet on a platform and hands on the floor, they'll be harder.
- Hold a 60-second plank. You can do this with your forearms or hands. If you're a beginner, place your hands on an elevated surface (chair, desk) and your feet on the floor; the angle will make the plank easier.

If you cannot do any of the above, make sure you do as much brisk walking as possible during the break. Most important is to utilize lunch hour by spending more time walking before or after lunch and not spending over time sitting at the lunch table chit chatting. You can chit-chat while walking together also.

Some Toys/gadgets for the Workouts

There are a good number of them available, but here are a few mentioned which can help in aiding you to do some exercises.

- **Powerball:** For arm toning, spin it for 1 to 2 minutes a few times a day.
- **Ankle weights:** Discreetly workout by strapping on some of these and doing a few under-desk leg lifts.
- **Egg-shaped hand exercise balls/normal sponge ball:** Squeezing these can help relieve tension and stress while strengthening your hands, wrists and forearms.

- **Resistance Bands:** You can workout your arms, chest, back and shoulders right at your desk. Resistance bands are portable.

As you spend the maximum amount of time inside the office, following some of the above-mentioned suggestions will certainly improve your level of fitness at office. These suggestions are increasingly important for your health as much as working hard is necessary for your career.

NINE

Second Quitter Syndrome

The results of your toil are finally becoming visible. You've started receiving compliments and you are brimming with confidence. You look good, you feel good, you have finally arrived. Certainly, you are an achiever. By now you are well-known as a fitness freak. You are getting used to appreciations from various quarters and you are very well aware that some folks are checking you out. If you go to any party, you might have received comments like, 'Oh! We are envious of your physique', 'What use is a life without food and free time'. Some comments are made in light humour, while others are made to tease you. If such barrages of comments are not enough, some close friends will wink, smile and say, 'What's the use of this fitness, if you are not using it properly, every investment has to have an ROI'. All these make you realize that fitness has become an important part your daily routine.

I am sure you will agree that quitting at this stage is simply foolish. But people do quit at this stage and surprisingly in sizeable numbers. So why do people quit after achieving so much? Let's look into some of the reasons:

Am I in a Good Shape? Can I Afford to Give Up?

'Isn't it that you are getting addicted to gyming?' commented my wife when I told her that I would accompany her to mall only after I finish my workout.

She replied, 'You are in good shape, now you can afford to miss a few days.' This statement was certainly the opposite of her earlier comment, 'Do something with your tummy', which propelled me towards fitness.

Skipping a few days or weeks certainly will not have much impact and you can afford it. As you are getting kudos for your new look and you come across as a confident person, you might reconsider skipping gym. According to FitnessForWeightLoss.com article 'Gym Statistics: Members, Equipment and Cancellations', the average gym member, not the fitness freaks, goes to the gym twice a week. So why feel guilty if you are skipping a few days?

This is the first question that comes to mind.

> **Caution** It starts with missing a few days in the week, then a full week of absence from the gym. Then it all depends upon the mood.

All our actions are based on how we have trained our brain. Nothing happens abruptly but then this mindset is the source of all ills. It is a fact that muscle grows in a rested body and we use this logic as an excuse to become irregular because if you surprise the body with exercise at some intervals, the impact will be more. If you justify being irregular at the gym, you are bound to enter into a trap. A day will come when you will really stop going to the gym. Initially, you will not feel anything missing because any adverse impact can be seen or felt only after a good number of weeks or few months, depending on person to person. Slowly, skipping gym becomes a norm and one day you will find that your fitness, for which you toiled so much, has taken a beating.

It requires a strong willpower to come back to a routine. After being regular to the gym for around six years, I have met many folks who were at a high level of fitness, but discontinued and came back after a good number of months.

One of them said, 'I could feel my paunch had started to show. That is why I came back.'

Then he quickly added, 'I am still fit in comparison to my friends and co-workers.'

The second statement is clearly an attempt to hide some type of guilt. I saw him for a few days and he disappeared again. I thought he might have changed his gym timing as people tend to do so, but then he reappeared again after a few weeks. This time, it was not in the gym but in a nearby grocery store and he was not the same what he was before.

'Are you still a regular at the gym?' he asked me and quickly added,

'Oh my god! You are still improving.'

He sheepishly smiled and said, 'I will come back. I have to get back in shape.'

I have not seen him again.

It is how you condition your mind. A little bit laxity here or irregularity there will not be an issue. But slowly, irregularity prolongs, forming a new habit of bunking the gym. One fine day, you will realize that you are not as fit as you used to be. Your tummy is not that flat anymore; pants have started to tighten. The same people who used to admire your fitness are now passing snide remarks.

'Didn't I tell you that it is very difficult to maintain, so why to try at all.'

Once you have worked so hard, how can you lose all your gains just by being complacent or taking things casually? Some people justify that if one can gain fitness once, then one can regain it at any time in future. This is partly correct, but then why to go through such pains. It is a fuelling mental agony when you have already reaped mental benefits of fitness and now you are giving them away.

> **Tip!** Have some friends who are into fitness: It is recommended that one has a buddy to start the gym, but then at this stage also there is a need for a buddy or someone in the fitness freak club to save one from quitting the gym.

The article 'Staying Healthy: Why Is Fitness Buddy Is All You Need' in *The Guardian* quotes Jeff Breckon, an exercise psychologist at Sheffield Hallam University, who said 'an exercise partner can work as a healthy competition or a role model who can get you out when you don't feel like it… It creates a sense of responsibility to someone else and social cohesion within a group of like-minded people.' He further says, 'If you just go on the treadmill or rower, time can feel like it is going very slowly. But if you're distracted, your perception of how much you are exerting yourself is much less. If you find that working out with someone is helping you to get fitter,' he adds, 'ask someone else to join, too, and pass on the positive contamination.'

The article further states that according to researchers at the Kansas State University, the trick of working out with someone who is fitter also makes sense. In one study, they found participants worked out for up to 200 per cent longer if they felt they were with someone who was better than they were.

> **Tip!** Fitness is a journey and, in this journey, set the next goal to avoid the feeling of quitting.

What next? Some people always look up to someone who is very fit, some of them maintain their fitness to keep inspiring others and act as their role models. Even if you are in great shape, you need to have a goal to maintain it and avoid taking your fitness lightly which will slowly lead you to the downward path. You need to be greedy and patient.

I have not yet faced this problem of quitting as I still feel there is enough room for improvement. Moreover, when I am publishing this book, how can I ever think about quitting?

Boredom

Boredom sets in due to the same schedule you follow in the gym. One of my friends asked me, 'How come you walk daily on the treadmill? Isn't it quite boring?' It was a fair question. As I walk on the treadmill almost at constant speed, it serves as the best time to reflect on important things that have happened throughout the day without getting distracted. Another friend commented on the monotony of using the treadmill.

> **Caution** Monotony plays an important role in quitting, but then don't we perform many daily duties which are monotonous. Still, we do them for the upkeep of our hygiene and body. Then why cannot we consider exercise also as something necessary for life.

It is true that exercises are somewhat same for months though there could be some daily variations. However, in order to get the desired result, the exercise has to be repetitive. Only when the body adjusts to an exercise and starts giving diminishing results, it is the time to change it.

The article '3 Ways to Avoid Boredom in the Gym' published in expertrain.com invites people to try these three tricks to avoid quitting the gym. To avoid monotony of treadmill or cycle, do a circuit training by using three machines—cross trainer, cycle and treadmill for 5 minutes each at the speed prescribed by your trainer and then repeat the cycle again with 4 minutes each and then for 3, 2 and finally 1 minute. The second way is to try a new machine or take up some other activity and the third one is to change your playlist so that music can break the monotony.

Boredom also happens when over time you start seeing fewer and fewer familiar faces with whom you had developed a bonding. This also starts to demotivate and add boredom to gym. Rather than feeling demotivated, you can take this as an opportunity to know new folks and it may be possible that some might become your new gym buddy, providing a new set of experience and suggestions.

> **Tip!** Every category of exercise has various options. Keep those options open and keep rotating them to avoid boredom. Make new friends in the gym and by changing trainers, you can get good suggestions which help in breaking the monotony.

Another cause of boredom is hitting the plateau at the gym. I have hit the plateau a good number of times but due to my long stint in the gym, I have worked with many trainers and most of them were not personal trainers, I used to change the exercise to see the result, which motivated me a lot. In addition, every trainer has different experiences and it is better to leverage that by changing them. My reason for changing trainers is actually due to attrition in the gym rather than a conscious choice. Still, a time came when I could not find any visible change over a year. I tried everything possible and then my trainer suggested taking inputs from the other trainer who had joined the gym recently and the new schedule started showing results. That has put a new dose of enthusiasm in gyming.

As in the initial days when my trainer used to call me to make sure I should not miss any session, similarly at this stage if you are feeling bored, you can request your gym manager or trainer, to give you a buzz from the gym. This could be for that period when you are under boredom. Recently, I came across one article validating this point on *Huffington Post* written by Toby Nwazor under the title '4 Reasons People Quit on Fitness Goal' and one of them is 'No Accountability or Consequences to Quitting'. The article states a study done by the Stanford University in 2010 to find just how important social support is, even if in small doses, which can help people trying to forge new fitness habits.

> In the study, 218 people were split into three groups: Those that would receive a call from a Stanford health educator every three weeks for a year, those that would receive a similar call but from a computer making human-like inquiries, and finally, those that would not receive any call monitoring their fitness progress. After 12 months, participants in the first group were exercising 178 minutes a week, more than the government-recommended 150 minutes. Participants in

the second group were above the fold as well, with 157 minutes a week. The third group, while still maintaining exercise habits, exercised 118 minutes a week. This means that it's easier to quit when we've only made a pact with ourselves, and thus have nobody else to disappoint.

> **Tip!** As self-discipline towards fitness is not a strong point for many, people tend to rely on social support not only in developing the habit but also in maintaining it.

Seeing the role of social influence on people's fitness outlook, there are many startups, which have flourished in the space of social fitness. Some of them revolve around an activity to make sure people attend physical activities like aerobics, Zumba, etc., while some other invite people to share their fitness vitals like number of steps taken in a day, calories intake, floors climbed, distance covered and so on, which put a social pressure on the lazy ones. There are gadgets too available too, which aid in social fitness in addition to their own individual tracking of fitness vitals.

It is also important to subscribe to get your daily dose of fitness videos and articles as news feed. This trick has really helped me. It raises the bar of fitness, encourages to try new things. The daily feed of stories, videos, diets keeps me motivated, challenged and if I miss or think of missing the gym, they make me feel guilty. It renews my determination to do it better the next day.

Everyone has a few set of clothes, which fit so well that they are worn multiple times and bring many positive nods and looks. Such clothes are also confidence enhancers.

When you start to go out of shape, look at these outfits and try them. It will prompt you to take corrective action immediately if you are not fitting well into them.

If nothing works, put placards, posters in your room or at your workplace, which will remind you of the pains you have gone through, and inspire you to carry on.

> **Tip!** Exercise videos on your cellphone, fitness quotes at workstations, good-fitting clothes in wardrobe and many such things will help in dragging you back to gym.

Changes in Personal Life or Daily Schedule

I have seen bachelors being regular to gym and suddenly after marriage, they disappear. Newly-married people have different priorities and attending a gym takes a back seat.

> **Tip!** Gym could be treated as a place for some quality time by the couple, and doing workout together will bond them better.

Another disruption happens when they enter parenthood. Even in such demanding times, you can certainly find time to do some exercises at least at home. It could be of shorter duration and a lesser frequency, but the habit should continue. Some of them take shorter breaks at work and utilize the time to attend office gym or to take brisk walking after lunch. You could maintain yourself in many ways.

Many youngsters, who were regular gymers in their college days, have to adjust to a new environment after getting a job. Some of them want to join the gym once they have settled, but then are unable to find time from the new job where they have to prove themselves. This is a feeling of guilt because you attend the gym without diluting any of your work commitment, as no job requires you to work forever, though there could be a phase of long hours. Most of the time citing work pressure is just another excuse to skip the gym.

> **Tip!** It is a myth that those who attend gym have lots of free time. Reality is that those who go to gym have a better sense of time management.

Then, there are some regulars to the gym but have to move to a new city. The same process of adjustments, settling into the new environment follows and their regular schedule takes a hit.

Another reason why people quit the gym is when their job function has changed or they have more responsibility at work, affecting their earlier schedule. It could also be a job change in the same city, where the office has different timings, a different route to work, etc., disrupting one's normal schedule.

There could be many personal and professional excuses for discontinuing the gym.

> **Tip!** Gyms have proliferated like anything. Every nook or corner has one. Offices and residential complexes have their own gyms. Excuse of not finding time to attend a gym is not true. There are exercises that could be done at home too.

Taking Alternatives to Gym

I would not call this quitting. You are quitting the gym, but you are not quitting fitness. I know some people who have left the gym and taken up some sports, yoga or marathon and started a new kind of fitness routine. All physical activities clubbed with a good diet leads to fitness. It is much more than just a display of muscles—to have core strength, body agility and so on. I conduced the first ever endurance test in my office and most of the exercises were floor based like plank, crunches, jumping jack, mountain climb, squats, etc., and those who focused on core strength training rather than pure bodybuilding took most of the awards. Certainly, if I conducted bodybuilding exercises, these folks would have won. On finding out what fitness regime those prize winners have undertaken, some of them have taken up gyming, others have taken a mix of bodybuilding regimes with one or two of activities like yoga, Zumba, Pilates, aerobics, etc., and some do home exercises and run marathons.

Some gyms also offer various classes and they suggest mixing such activities in addition to regular gyming for better results.

You can take up such activities if you are disciplined. I have heard people say that they switched gyms with some sports, and on digging into this further, I found out that they are not regulars in their new activities. Some of them joined swimming but stopped, as the weather was not favourable. Some of them started to go for badminton or tennis, but then stopped as the partner with whom they played was not able to join. Marathon runners focus only a few days before the event, as marathons don't happen every day.

> **Tip!** Any activity or a mix of activity, which one is unable to undertake at least 3-4 times a week, should be supplemented with exercise in gym or home for the rest of the week to maintain fitness.

Such mix of activities enables you to keep fit. This will also help you do better in your sports or other activities, which you have just substituted with full-time gym and reduce the chances of injury too.

Medical Injuries

For those who love to exercise and maintain their fitness, any injury, which will make them rest for some time, is a punishment. Even a thought of not attending the gym, is quite demotivating for such people. It is common to see such people haggle with their doctor to allow them to attend the gym earlier than prescribed. Some folks are in a weight-loss programme and are concerned that everything they have achieved might be negated due to this injury. While someone who has bulked up but did not get time to cut down on their weight feels frustrated with such a thought. Then, there are some others who have been initiated into fitness with a lot of coercing and are now worried that such a prolonged inaction will wean away their motivation and will power, and most likely will keep them away from gym forever.

If you face some injury and are asked to rest for a good number of weeks or months, how will you handle it?

Let us focus on what happens to your body when you stop going to the gym. Here I mean 'stop' is not just a pause for a couple of weeks, but a long one. Take solace that you will not become unfit or get out of shape immediately. As fitness is a slow process, where body takes time to react, similarly the reverse is also true.

In the article 'What Happens If You Stop Going to Gym' written by Ryn Gargulinski published in livestrong.com says that:

> Your cardiovascular fitness level declines when you stop your aerobic workouts. Highly trained athletes, for instance, experience a rapid and dramatic decline in their cardiovascular fitness for the first three weeks after they stop working out, after which time the fitness loss slows down, according to the American Council on Exercise. If your level of fitness is high, but lower than a pro-athlete, your fitness level will start to drop after about 12 weeks. If your fitness level is low to moderate, you'll only retain your fitness level for a few weeks, after which it will decline quickly. Your muscular strength declines when you give up your strength training routine, depending on your level of fitness and how long you've been strength training. Highly trained athletes can expect to retain their muscular strength for several weeks or even months. They will also maintain a higher level of fitness after they stop lifting weights than those who are newer to strength training. If you're new to strength training, your muscles atrophy at a quicker rate and can regress to the same level they were before you began your strength training routine.

People should certainly try to do whatever they can, depending upon the type of injury to make sure they remain fit. I have come across a person in my gym, who had got his left arm in a cast and he was doing leg exercises and other exercises like lifting dumbbells from the other arm. I thought this would have been a one off case where this person is dedicated to fitness, but then I came across an article '7 Ways to Maintain Muscle When You are Not Working Out' published on thefitnessmagazine.com written by Carey Rossi, suggested exercising the rest of your (non-injured) body. 'If your left leg is injured, for example, there's benefit to training the uninjured leg,' says David Hooper, MS, CSCS, a graduate research assistant in the Ohio State University College of Education and Human Ecology in this article. He further says, 'It has been shown to transfer to the injured limb to some degree.' Yes, exercising one part of your body can help maintain the muscle in other parts—crazy, right?

My respect for such people is certainly very high.

> **Tip!** Most of the people, who are forced into fitness are the ones who escape with the first sign of injury. Please continue to exercise with the uninjured part of the body.

Fitness is part of your lifestyle, even though everyone wants to be injury free, one can get injured outside or inside the gym. Find out what you can do during injury without aggravating it. You must take inputs from your doctor and accordingly make plan during your injuries.

So, what will happen to muscles which you have built over time. Will it all go away? Will favourite shirts not be that fit. One other article 'How to Maintain Muscle When You're Injured and Not Working Out' in aworkoutroutine.com talks about taking care of muscles during injuries. It says that those who want to maintain muscle during an injury period when their physical activity is abysmally low, can take a few things which are mentioned in the article. It makes sense to preserve muscle by keeping the protein intake high. But this alone may not be sufficient. One tends to put on weight fast when they are rested for long time because their normal calorie intake is at the level where physical activity is high. It is important to have calorie intake, which will keep you in maintenance mode.

Another thing that the article mentioned is that one needs to maintain the good habits like getting plenty of sleep, drinking plenty of water and taking sufficient amount of nutrition, etc., to keep your body in good shape. Muscle memory is real, and the author mentioned that he was out of action for three months and when he came back from injury, regaining muscle was quite fast.

When not attending gym, continue to watch fitness videos, read fitness articles and eat wisely to ensure that not much is lost during your resting period. It is certainly good news that any temporary setback in fitness schedule will not cause many problems, but then one has to come back to fitness regime. After achieving so much, quitting at this stage is certainly not a wise decision.

TEN

Make Fitness Your Lifestyle

Journey of fitness is like any other journey. This also has its highs and lows, happiness and setbacks, results and plateaus, excitement and boredom and much more. Despite all the twists and turns that someone experiences in this journey, he or she can vouch for the change it has brought in their professional and personal life.

So why cannot you make it a part of your life? Why cannot you make it a part of your daily schedule?

Certainly, you can!

After all, why do you brush your teeth daily? Why do you take shower daily and sometimes twice a day? Umm, it is because it is good for your hygiene. Similarly, after knowing all the benefits that fitness can bring in your lifestyle, it is important that you continue with this journey of fitness and make it a part of your lifestyle just as you do with other basic habits of hygiene.

Recently, I was visiting San Francisco for an event at the company where my daughter was interning. There were other parents too. Since there was some time for the event to start, my daughter took me around the premises, when she got a message. She read it and started laughing.

'I do not want to tell you, because it will go to your head,' she told me.

But she could not hold her excitement and blurted it out, 'My other intern friend texted me that your dad looks very cool. Your fitness is making waves here too.'

I feel proud that making fitness as a part of my lifestyle is influencing the next generation too. Both my son and daughter are very particular about their fitness. My wife who used to do yoga has joined my gym and added aerobics as well to her routine. A sense of pride and satisfaction certainly comes when you see your family has also embraced fitness and made it a part of their lifestyle.

I wanted to test my fitness and was looking for some new avenues to test. I had never been in a stageshow even during my school days. During our office's annual family gala evening event, I could not say no to the request to come on stage. I performed a five-minute long dance medley with my employees which was well-choreographed and required a huge effort during the practice sessions. At this stage of my life, I was entering into a territory mostly reserved for people half my age, performing in front of thousand people was a toast to fitness.

Can We Make Fitness a Contagious Habit?

When a person my age takes up fitness, it makes a huge impact on employees. Membership in office gym has swelled. Unlike many other initiatives, which die slowly, yoga classes continued year after year. Registrations in company-sponsored marathons are increasing year after year.

Something interesting happened a while back at my workplace. Anyone who wants to take an internal transfer to any management role has to go through an internal screening process. I also meet such candidates to ascertain their suitability.

One person came for such a screening. He was sitting quite stiffly for long with his arms folded, covering his tummy. It was seemed awkward; I thought he would be nervous, so I asked him, 'Please sit comfortably so that we can enjoy the conversation.'

He stiffened further. I was puzzled but kept quiet. He sensed that I was uncomfortable and sheepishly looked down and said, 'My colleagues have warned me that if you see my tummy, you will reject me.'

I split into laughter and assured him that such a thing will not happen, but then I advised him to take up fitness.

I have completed six years in fitness and can easily claim that anyone can be fit by following most of the suggestions recommended in this book. It is our right to be fit. It is in the interest of our society to spread the message of fitness. If each one of us can spread this fitness fever, we can bring on a revolution, where medical bills will reduce, productivity at work will increase, longevity will become a blessing and an immense satisfaction will be achieved by influencing others' lives in a positive way.

The famous book *Sapiens: A Brief History of Humankind*, written by Yuval Noah Harari has captured the changes in the life of Homo sapiens. Homo sapiens continued to live by gathering wild plants and hunting wild animals, which changed more than 10,000 years ago when they usurped agricultural revolution and devoted time and effort in manipulating lives of many animals and plant species. The author further said that in the last 500 years, a permanent revolution took place, called the industrial revolution, which started to convert our blue and green planet into concrete and plastic heaps.

In current times, don't you agree that the speed at which technology is evolving is increasing with every passing time and forcing us to become more sedentary? As contrasted to being so active in the jungle to gather wild plants and hunt for animals, food is now just a click away and we are comfortably eating in our homes. Though our body has adapted to some of the changes but this adaptation is still slower than the way we have changed our way of living. We still take nine months to deliver a baby. So, it is important to listen to the basics of our body and become active in our daily life. As the speed of technological changes will only increase, a need for fitness revolution is certainly justified.

This revolution can only be successful when each one of us becomes a role model of fitness for people who in turn can become role models for others.

Let us not procrastinate, wake up and commit yourself to fitness.

Acknowledgments

My journey towards fitness has been shaped by many at various stages in my life. I have tried to thank as many of them, but please accept my apologies if I have missed anyone out inadvertently.

First, I would like to thank my son, Utsav, who drew my attention to my growing paunch with grave concern. However, I did not seriously begin to introspect the issue until my wife, Deepti, expressed her worries about my physical and physiological changes. So when my colleague Mohit Misra, shared his experience of how a new set of trousers in the mall were not looking good on him and he wanted to hit the gym, the thought struck a chord with me.

Pramodh Kumar, my personal trainer, whose persistence and persuasion to the extent that he made my goal towards achieving fitness his own, enabled me to stick to the regime despite the initial painful period when the results were hardly visible. My gym physiotherapist Rosmi Abey, manager Brajesh Kumar and trainer Mukesh Sahu assisted me as well. Though I learnt a lot from many gym members, Harsh Ranjan and Ravi Ranjan deserve a special mention.

During my journey of fitness, one person who always stood by me and assured me that I am on the right track is my general physician Dr C.M.A. Beliappa. His support doubled my enthusiasm to continue to achieve new heights.

My daughter Vidushi, who saw the first draft of the book and suggested valuable changes to ensure that the book strike the right chord with readers. Lohith Shivaram, my colleague, helped immensely during this journey by providing wise tips and suggestions whenever I was in a dilemma. He, together with Sandeep Shetty and Sharat Wodeyar, have reviewed each and every line of this book and also provided wider perspectives to some sections based on their own experiences. Lohith and Sandeep have also contributed some portions on gym exercises.

Ardent follower of fitness, Tom Fallon, CEO of Infinera, has continuously motivated me during this journey. I also gained knowledge from some colleagues, Syed Aasimuddin, Navin Rajan, Saurabh Pandey, Vishal Arhatia, Payal Madan, Puneet Pandita, Dharmendra Kalita, Prakash Bisht and Ritu Raj, who are fitness enthusiasts as well. A steady flow of positive feedback from Kirti Naidu helped me too. Jaya Johnson's advice on book format and type of sections to be covered by experts was very apt.

The book would not have been complete without the help of fitness experts and their contributions for the special sections in it. Thanks to Vinod Channa, Ash Nath, Rashmi Cherian, Luvena Rangel together with Pradeep Gowda, Shweta Mehta and Gopakumar S.

Dibakar Ghosh of Rupa Publications and I worked together not only on the idea of the book, but every step of the way. Lastly, a big thanks to Anurupa Sen for putting in long hours during editing to give the book its final shape.